william
absolutely uninvited

mandy duggan

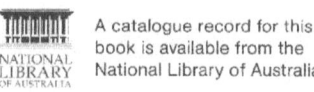 A catalogue record for this book is available from the National Library of Australia

Copyright © 2021 Mandy Duggan
All rights reserved.
ISBN-13: 978-1-922343-64-2

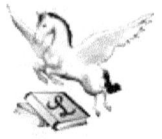

Linellen Press
265 Boomerang Road
Oldbury, Western Australia
www.linellenpress.com.au

Dedication

With gratitude to the loves of my life, my children, Neesha and Josh. You have shown me a love like no other, and given me the fortitude to dig deeper when I thought I had hit rock bottom, and the courage to speak my own truth, even if that means I stand alone.

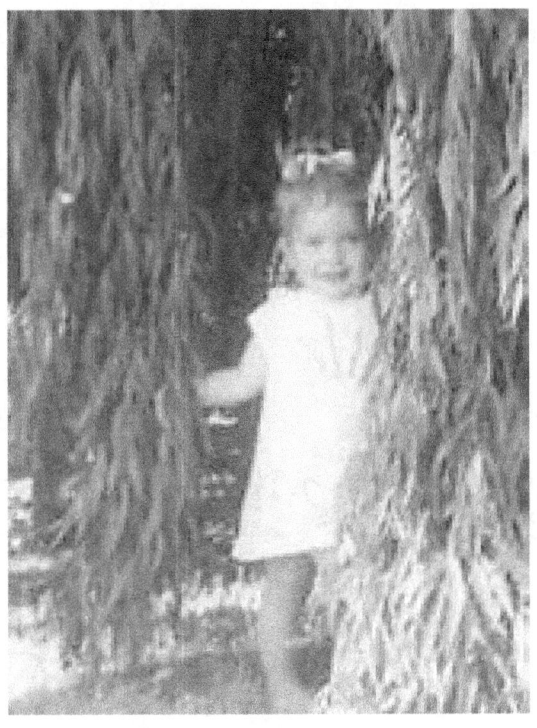

Cover photograph Mandy Duggan age two years.

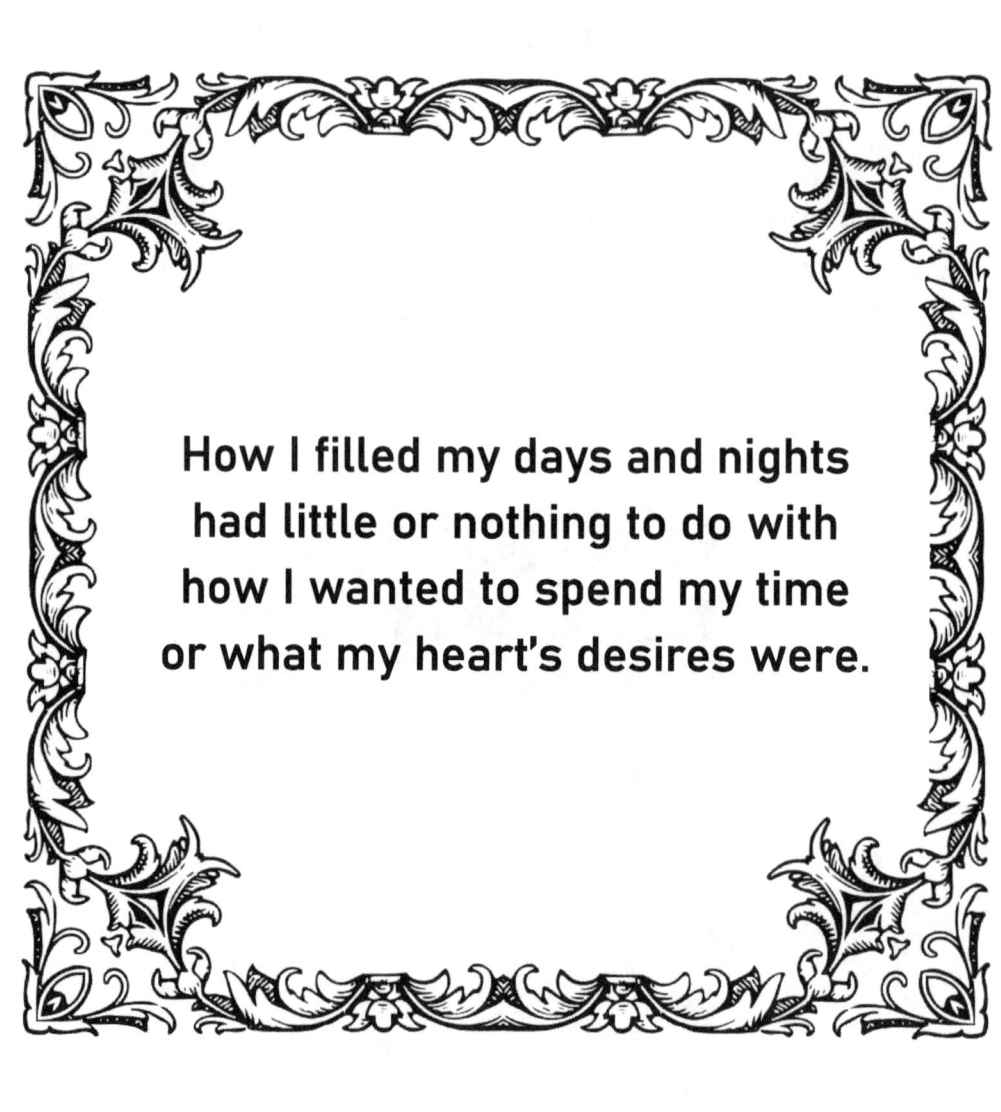

How I filled my days and nights had little or nothing to do with how I wanted to spend my time or what my heart's desires were.

just begin

I snuggled alongside my mother last night. In the early hours of this morning, she laid her hand on mine and stroked her thumb across my hand. The warmth of her touch radiated up my arm and into my heart. This simple gesture made me realise just how much I have ached for this contact with my mum and reminded me that I am loved by her.

I had become so busy with life that I lost sight of the value of connection with those I love. That is, I did not realise just how disconnected I had become; how isolated I had become until cancer came crashing into my world and I fell down the rabbit hole.

Life was a myriad of demands on my time. How I filled my days and nights had little or nothing to do with how I wanted to spend my time or what my heart's desires were. My mornings would be a typical blur of cramming exercise in before the sun came up, preparing school lunches, getting kids out of bed, going to work and chasing my tail all day long, before rushing out the door to do school pick up and after school activities (sports training etc.); dropping off to work, or friend's places, picking up, washing, cleaning, making beds, preparing meals and squeezing in some socialising when I could manage it.

I can't remember the last time I didn't feel exhausted. In fact, I became so adept at not feeling that it made it much easier to keep going with this ridiculously busy, selfless lifestyle – something I now refer to as the 'daily grind' period of my life journey.

My heart is open now and I feel everything, allowing me to move through every experience with love. Even if I am afraid or sad.

I'm sitting under my patio at the moment, in a rare afternoon of winter sunshine. A noisy flock of birds is making a racket and the thought of impending rain comes to mind. I hear a plane overhead as well and I fleetingly wonder how divine the world would look from the sky.

I need to write my story to express and there is so much to say that the words are tripping over one another in my mind and blocking the stairwell to my creative expression. It's been like this for some time now: Me knowing that I need to write my story – get it out of my body – but unable to pull consecutive words from the mountains that have been piling up these past four years.

So I've decided to just "begin". How good that word feels.

Begin

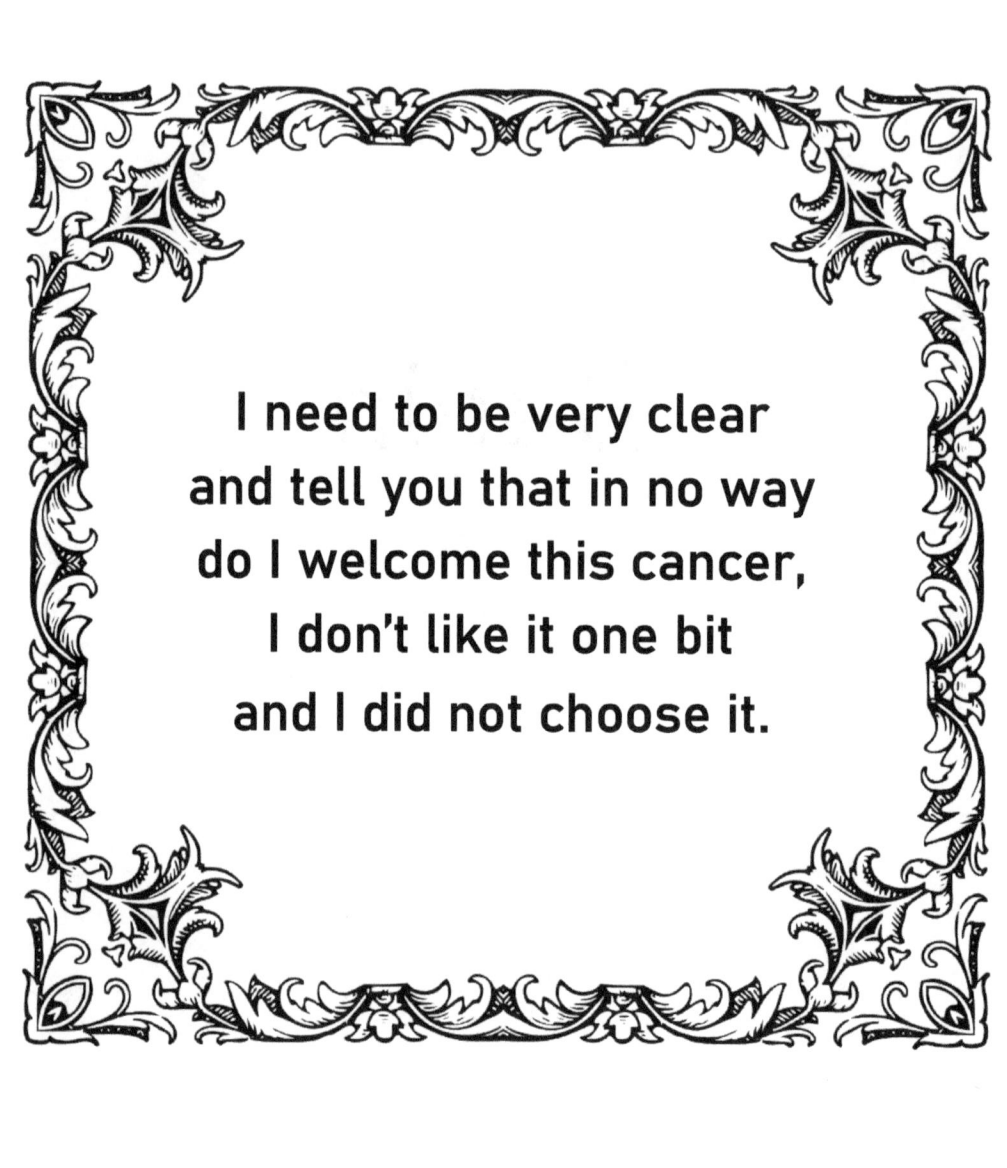

I need to be very clear
and tell you that in no way
do I welcome this cancer,
I don't like it one bit
and I did not choose it.

introducing William

(absolutely uninvited)

William came crashing through the ether and into my life on 3 April 2014, one of those moments that I have not been able to *unremember*. Time really does slow down and there is a lag between the movement of your doctor's mouth and the sound of the words reaching your ears. When you are told that you have cancer, this really does happen. My mind went into absolute fear and I have spent most of the time since absolutely terrified.

I don't intend to relive the experiences that unfolded from that time in great detail here, other than to say: I hope that I never have to go through a bone marrow biopsy again. *Ever*. This was an extremely traumatic experience for me that I can only describe as similar to having a cork screw wound down through your flesh, tissue and bone and into the marrow. Although I didn't feel pain, I felt the pressure and force of that horrid little instrument going through my body and I wanted to run away every second of every minute. The only thing stopping me from wishing it wasn't me lying there was the thought that it would be someone else.

I was formally diagnosed as having a malignant blood condition on 13 May 2014 and at that time the diagnosis was *Macroglobulinaemia*. The bone marrow biopsy was necessary to determine the specific subtype and this was carried out on 10 June 2014. Three and half weeks later – which was actually an eternity spent waiting for a cancer diagnosis.

I received a letter from my haematologist confirming *Waldenstrom's Macroglobulinaemia*.

Acronym: WM   AKA: William (absolutely uninvited).

I will never refer to William (absolutely uninvited) without the 'absolutely uninvited'. Although I have been able to become more accepting of the diagnosis, I need to be very clear and tell you that in no way do I welcome this cancer, I don't like it one bit and I did not choose it.

William (absolutely uninvited) is a rare and incurable type of *Non-Hodgkin's lymphoma*. The incurable part was something that I blatantly refused to accept initially, and I spent at least two years insisting there is no such thing as incurable and believing that I could banish it from my body by the sheer force of my will.

And in those years, I would be so hopeful at blood test time, using all of my might to manifest miraculous results that announced no sign of paraprotein, no high IgM, no low IgG, no high ESR and no indication of William (absolutely uninvited). And the doctors would be astounded and I would live happily ever after.

The crashing despondence that I felt each time those blood results confirmed that William (absolutely uninvited) had not miraculously disappeared and that I was not cancer free created such a low for me.

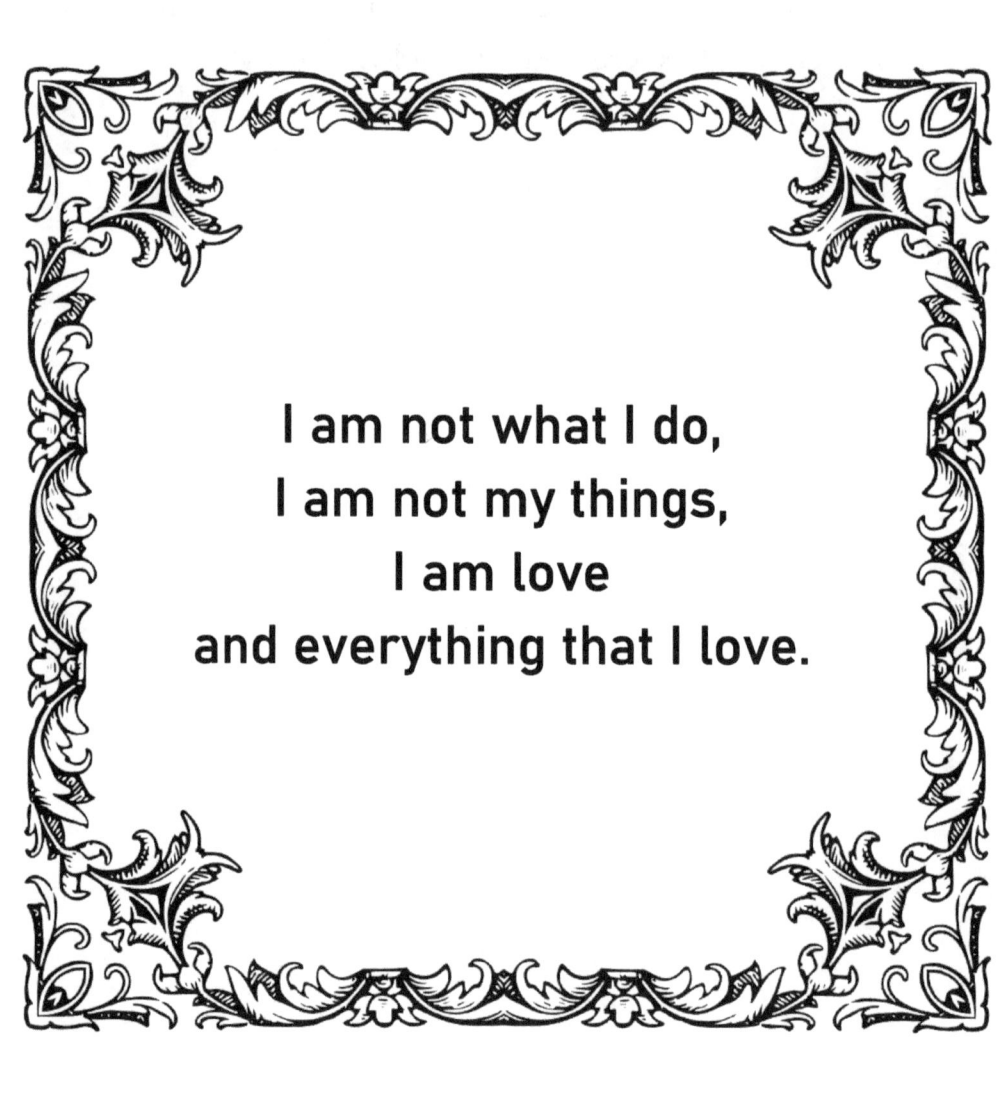

I am not what I do,
I am not my things,
I am love
and everything that I love.

discovering mandy

As I floundered in the early days – post-diagnosis I tried to come up with a plan to give William (absolutely uninvited) the fight of his very existence – I was completely overwhelmed. I knew how important this would be to my recovery and yet I just didn't know where to start; what to focus on first. I was inundated with no end of information about miracle cures, pills, plants, drinks, potions; all claiming to be the miracle cure of cancer. I was very unwell, extremely fatigued and completely terrified.

People around me reacted to the news, each in their own way. My circle of people was quite large initially, but soon reduced to the people I knew I could lean on when I needed to and be however I was in any given moment.

What I did learn very quickly is that most people either didn't know how to respond to the diagnosis or felt that I needed to just get back to work and back into the busy routine of my life and I would be fine. I felt like they were speaking a foreign language.

I couldn't take my eyes off my kids; I wanted to drink in as much of them as possible, as if each time I hugged them or looked at them or took in their essence was the last.

I grieved for their weddings that I would not attend; the grandchildren I wouldn't meet; the times when they needed me and I would not be there for them.

Rabbit hole, right?

In the midst of all this chaos and desperation, I was having a conversation with a dear friend telling her about my quest to know myself and she asked me "SO WHO ARE YOU?" I had no idea. Imagine that? I had no idea who I was.

Want to know?

Let's find Mandy!

And just like that, I had the starting point to my recovery. I realised I could not make a plan of self-recovery if I did not know who I was.

And so began my search for Mandy.

You see, I haven't been having a holiday full of frivolity. I've been climbing mountains, looking under rocks, inside crevices, listening to the wind.

I've connected with various healers to help me along the way: Life coaching, life alignment, kinesiology, Bowen therapy, massage, reflexology, meditation, crystals, harp healing, DoTerra Oils, crystal bed chakra healing, energy balance, all of which have helped me to discover myself and process how I feel about William showing up absolutely uninvited.

I've been spending time in nature almost every day, either sitting on the beach with my feet in the sand or in my back yard with the trees and the birds – just me and my soul.

I love it when my feet are planted in beach sand and I can sit and watch the ocean and smell and hear it. I've had the luxury of doing this for as long as I need to and as often as I like.

Solaris Cancer Care has been a sanctuary for me. As soon as I step inside, I am enveloped with loving and caring energy. Everyone who goes there is fighting the cancer battle, with such calm and determination and courage.

Who is Mandy?

I AM NOT WHAT I DO.

I am not my job
I am not a gardener
I am not a house cleaner, I am not a cook

I AM NOT MY THINGS
I am not the size of my house
or the suburb in which I live
I'm not the couch that I sit upon
I am not the size of my bling
I'm not who I'm married to

I am not the car that I drive
I'm not what's in my bank account
or the money in my purse
I am not the clothing that I wear
or how I wear my hair
I'm not the label of my handbag
or the make of my shoes
I'm none of these things, that's not who I am

I have been filling my days and nights for so long, I had completely lost any sense of who I am. Perhaps I have never really known myself.

I had to completely stop doing and just BE to find me.

I AM LOVE … And I am everything that I love.

I am the morning sun that lights up my garden
and creates diamonds upon the ocean
and sparkles in the reticulation

I am the bird orchestra that greets me in the morning
and chatters to me all day long
I am the miracles that I see every day
I am the breeze in my hair and on my skin
I am the cool beach sand on my feet
I am laughter that dances upon the wind
I am a hug for a friend with no words – just light
I am my newborn children snuggled
into my chest for the very first time
I am music and dancing and the words of a song

I'm an acoustic guitar and the strings of a harp

I am the tear in an eye
when something touches my heart
I'm friends around a table, all talking at once
I am courage and bravery and 100% heart
I am the sunset that colours the sky,
slips into the ocean with an evening sigh
I am the stars in the midnight sky
I'm the moonlight on my window
and the moon way up high

I'm rainbows and raindrops,
I'm snowflakes on windowsills
I'm sunflowers and rosebuds,
bees and butterflies
I'm a smile and I'm kindness,
I'm a gentle touch

I had to completely stop doing and just **BE** to find me.

I am energy and light and all of the above.

I am free to be me.

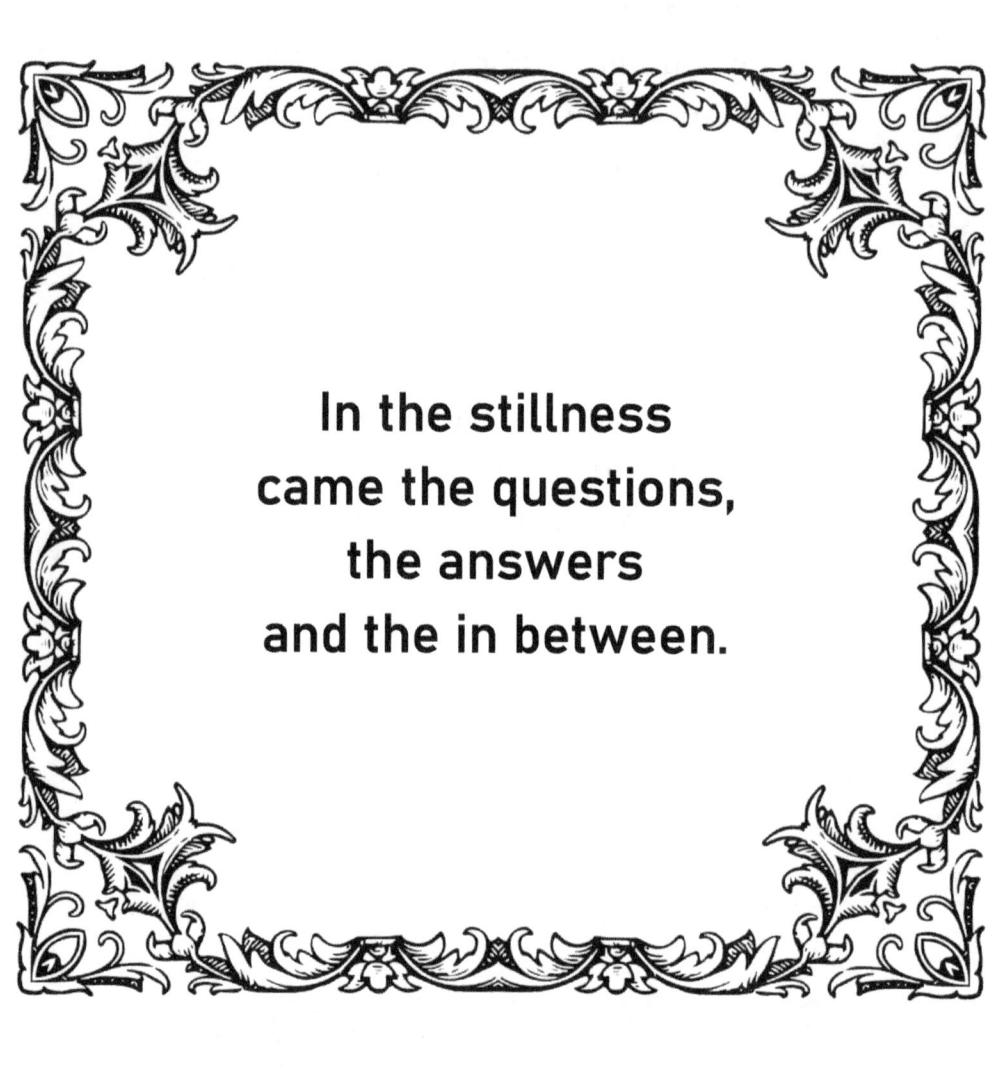

In the stillness
came the questions,
the answers
and the in between.

inwards

So began my journey inwards.

The plan went out the window by the way. Putting together a plan, that was *doing* not *being*.

It turns out, all I needed to do was start and let it all unfold.

I felt such a mess in my mind and my body and I really wasn't confident that listening to my intuition was what was right for me. I felt completely lost and so very afraid for years. Now, four years on, I know absolutely that I knew what I needed, no matter how chaotic that seemed at the time.

So there I was, unwell, terrified, severely anxious and having PTSD triggers left, right and centre.

I had spent most of my life until that point structuring my time, over-committing my energy and being an absolute control freak. Falling down the rabbit hole, trying desperately to find a foothold, I knew that I must let go of structure, stop doing and just let myself be still.

In the stillness came the questions, the answers and the in between.

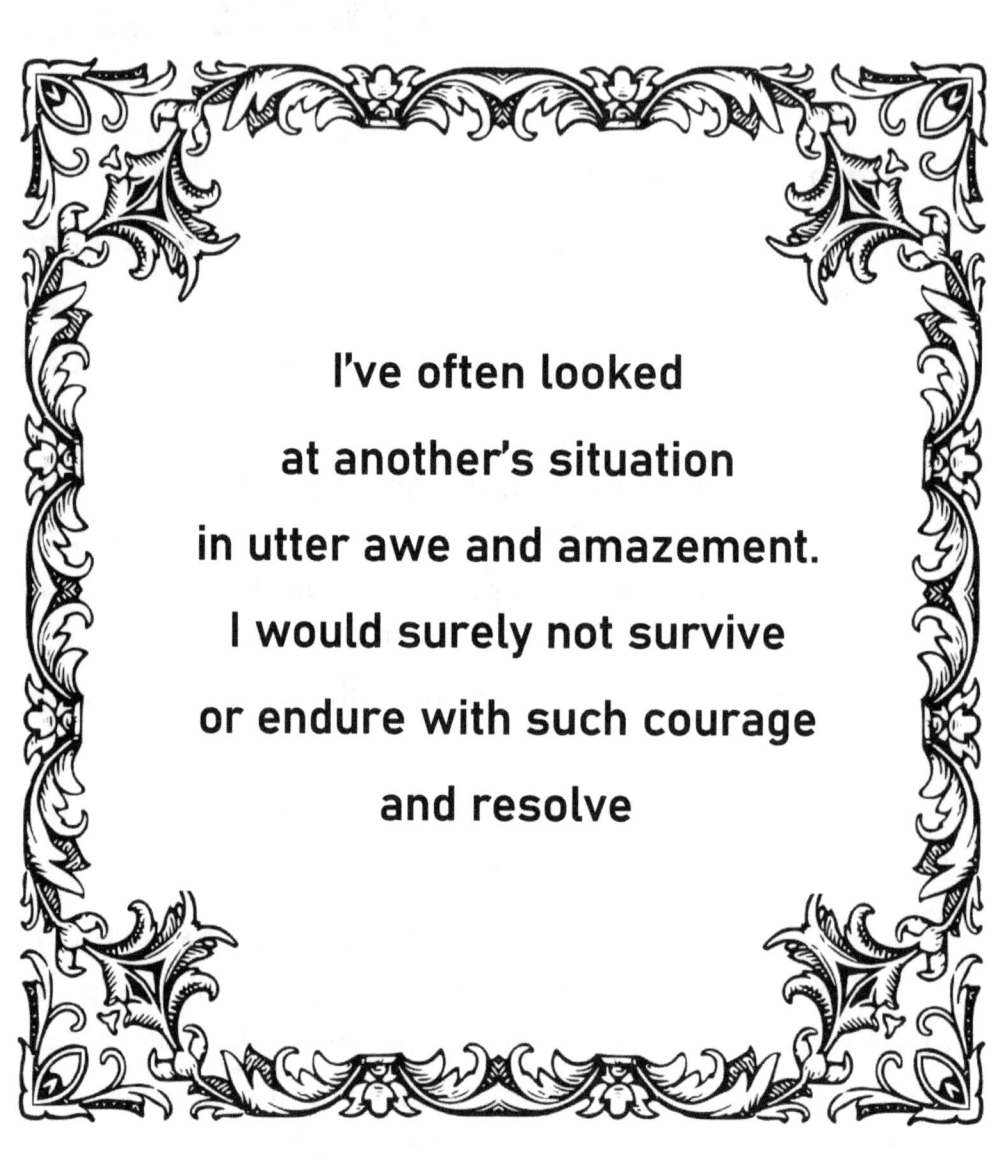

I've often looked
at another's situation
in utter awe and amazement.
I would surely not survive
or endure with such courage
and resolve

intrepid moments

I've met many people who have inspired me. I've often looked at another's situation in utter awe and amazement. I would surely not survive or endure with such courage and resolve. This inspiration has come out to hold my hand and prod me along at times, when my brain couldn't get the message to my body for me to act.

Ironically, I'd never been on a roller coaster ride until William came crashing into my life; absolutely uninvited. I avoided anything that would bring the contents of my stomach rushing toward my mouth.

When I stepped into the ED on the 20th of March 2014, I joined the queue and handed over my token, unwittingly boarding the South West Health Campus Ride of your Life! On the 17th of November 2014, I stepped off the crazy train and started to breathe big, gulping lungs-full of oxygen. I began seven weeks sick leave from my work, a time during which I slept a lot and started to realise that continuing to work was going to be a problem for me.

I remember thinking, "What the fuck am I going to do

with this? What the fuck am I going to do? YOU ARE GOING TO STOP DOING!"

> *Sometimes it's important to work for that pot of gold. But other times it's essential to take time off and to make sure that your most important decision in the day simply consists of choosing which colour to slide down on the rainbow*
>
> Douglas Pagels 2003

Bad movie, living nightmare, moments peppered with friendship skyscrapers, sparkles, unicorns and fields of sunflowers that must be revisited to bring me to a point of acceptance, healing and defragmentation:

20 MARCH 2014
- blood pressure 220/115 (ED)
- haemoglobin 80, 4 units of blood missing (ED)
- chronically anaemic (ED)

21 MARCH
Diagnosis: bursitis in right elbow, hypertension and anaemia (ED)

25 MARCH
"I need to carry out more blood tests, I'm worried that you have stopped producing blood" (GP)

3 APRIL
"You have a raised ESR level and an abnormal protein. You have cancer, I think it's bone marrow cancer. You need to have a bone marrow biopsy as soon as possible (GP)
You need to go back to hospital – you're very sick" (GP)

3-10 APRIL
In hospital

6 APRIL
Endoscopy and colonoscopy

8 APRIL
Intravenous iron infusion

10 APRIL
Diagnosis: MGUS (monoclonal gammopathy of unknown significance)
Additional comments: further investigation for multiple myeloma

13 MAY
Diagnosis: macrogobulinemia (suspected Waldenstrom's Macroglobulinemia)
Additional comments: bone marrow biopsy required to specifically diagnose type of blood cancer and determine next steps.

14 MAY
CT scan

10 JUNE
Bone marrow biopsy

26 JUNE
Phone information: no treatment required, early stages of disease

4 JULY
Written diagnosis: Waldenstrom's Macroglobulinemia

9 JULY
Ultrasound

25 NOVEMBER
Hysteroscopy

FEBRUARY 2015
Endometrial Novosure Ablation

Words that did not belong before, that I'm now complacent about (in no particular order): Haemoglobin, cannula, hypertension, light kappa chains, ESR, immunoglobulin (IgM), paraprotein, MGUS, multiple myeloma, Waldenstrom's Macroglobulinemia, marrow infiltration, bone marrow aspiration, bone trephine biopsy, hyperviscosity, bursitis, endoscopy, colonoscopy, hysteroscopy, intravenous iron infusion, ferritin, lymphocytes, platelets, deep vein thrombosis, mycrocitic, Bence Jones urine testing, immunosuppressed.

Those intrepid moments:

On the 3rd of April, I was standing in my GP of 20 years' room, watching her mouth the words "I've just received some results that show you have an elevated ESR and other things –I'm pretty sure you have cancer, bone marrow cancer. This is not a diagnosis, but I promise I will go through this with you and I will be honest with you."

The fight, flight or freeze chemical ignited in my brain and I went home, had a cup of tea and packed a bag to take to hospital; arranged for my son to get to his haircut, called my daughter, my mother, my employer and my best friend.

Somewhere between opening the front door and trying to find my overnight bag, finding a moment when my son was out of the room, I sobbed. I gasped for air at the same time, while my friend held me and cried along with me – just a couple of minutes of exposing what was going on inside of me. I heard my son approaching and wiped my eyes; pulled back my shoulders and stuffed that terror back down! Closing the top of my head with a *thud!* I asked if he needed a snack while handing him some money for his haircut.

The same day, but late that night I was alone and laying in a hospital bed when the emotional tsunami hit and I experienced my first panic attack. I met myself, the stripped away version – with this core of strength that got me through one of the longest nights of my life. I now know the value of existing one second a time and the value of the affirmation "right here, right now, I am okay". I said this in my mind over and over through the night to keep the terror from consuming me. I said this in my mind every time I felt the panic rising within me and I continue to do so.

On the 13th of May, I arrived at a quaint little home converted into medical rooms for an appointment with my haematologist. On the walk from the car park, I delighted in the homeliness of the front garden and precise pathway to the entrance of what I fondly referred to as Raven's Cottage – well, not so fondly, in fact, not fondly at all.

I had optimistically decided that my first meeting was going to clear up this bungled mess with an explanation that my results were confused with someone else's and it had all been a total comedy of errors. My bestie by my side, our mood was light. We had this.

Introducing himself with *"they call me Doctor Death"* wasn't exactly endearing. *"what the fuck!"*, came to mind. My heart may have shrieked to a grinding halt at the very same time as my brain when the doctor said to me, *"You have a malignant condition"*. The only physical awareness I recall was my best friend holding my hand and squeezing at the precise moment that I lost brain function. My hopes sunk to the pit of my stomach and I wanted to vomit.

And with that, William arrived. Absolutely uninvited.

On 10 June, I arrived at Raven's Cottage for a bone marrow biopsy with my bestie by my side. I noticed the gardens and the pathway on the other side of my shallow breathing with the affirmation *right here, right now you are okay* on continuous play in my mind.

In summary:

- it was not painful! it was traumatic
- it was the longest 10 minutes ever
- I will never look at a corkscrew in the same light
- I intend to never have another bone marrow biopsy.

I got through that experience with my trusty affirmation reciting in my mind, non-stop and my bestie holding my right foot.

Afterwards, we went to the Dome for a hot chocolate in a somewhat stunned state of shock, before collecting my son from school.

The next day, during a bone marrow biopsy debrief over the phone with my bestie, I asked if she was okay and she said to me, "Well, he was lucky he finished when he did, because I was just about to tell him that if he hurt my BFF any more, I would tackle him to the ground."

I started to laugh from the depths of my belly: 70% joy and 30% hysteria as I told my bestie that she hadn't thought that – she had said it out loud! She said it to the doctor as he announced that the biopsy was at an end with a hand on my shoulder, and told me that I had done really well.

We laughed and laughed to the point of tears.

Intrepid moments indeed.

At these times, I felt afraid and weak, not brave or courageous at all. On reflection, I can understand that I was at my strongest; the courage tank was low because I needed lots to get me through.

I say it, think it,
dodge it, hear it,
perhaps more than
any other word
and I've only just realised this.
The light bulb moment.
Enough has been there,
through every twist
and every turn.

enough

Enough? This little word really is the proverbial can of worms. Give a girl some time out to be alone with her thoughts and everything is possible!

Enough? This little word is so amazingly connected to human-ness that I can't type this quickly enough. Pun intended!

Enough.

Just pause a moment. What does it mean to you?

It's been the driving force for me throughout my life. Under every rock, in every shadow and in my healing too. Enough has shown up at every opportunity.

It's sat down with me for every meal.

It lurked through my childhood and low self-esteem moments.

It sat quietly and unobserved in my hospital room when I was broken and bruised in a car wreck.

It has stepped out of the ruins of my marriage, dusted itself off, held out its hand and helped me to my feet.

Enough co-parented with me and came to the rescue many a time in those sleep-deprived, train wreck moments.

It came home silently with me every day from my job, sitting upright and proud in the passenger seat, on a Friday night. If I was too tired, enough drove me home.

Enough.

I say it, think it, dodge it, hear it, perhaps more than any other word and I've only just realised this – the lightbulb moment – Enough has been there through every twist and turn.

William showing up – absolutely uninvited as you know – has been a catalyst for a questioning that can only happen when confronted with something so huge that you don't instantly bounce back, you don't get up, you flounder in dumbfounded-ness of proportions that you cannot conceive. When your mind reboots – I'm talking, after the three months of very little brain function whilst on auto pilot and the ensuing five months of denial and rapid construction of Mandy playing the lead role in MY LIFE IS NORMAL. THIS DIDN'T REALLY HAPPEN – and you face this thing head-on. Enough lingers dutifully as always.

It's amazing what you notice when you stop *doing* and just *be*. No easy feat for me, to just *be*. A soul that gasped for air whenever my head broke the surface of a furious whitewash of an alcoholic, child-bashing parent, oily alcoholic predators who interfered with the children unfortunate enough to be stuck in the same boiling pot. I stepped out of a childhood that resembled the pages of a Stephen King novel with only a crumb of self-worth and the resounding echo of ENOUGH!

From a place of *being* I can clearly see the road I've travelled and how "enough" would race ahead and jump out at me at every corner. When William showed up – absolutely uninvited – I was 20 years into a 22-year plan. The sweet smell of reclaiming my life when my children were both adults, was wafting like the smell of a freshly baked cake. The formula for this plan was basic. If I work hard *enough*. If I put *enough* time and effort into raising my children. If I am *enough*. Enough, enough, enough!

Enough ran rife through those years. Incessantly raving: You haven't eaten *enough* of your dinner. I've had *enough*! I don't have *enough* money to buy you that. I said *enough*! I'm not good *enough*.

What has been like a slap in the face with a wet fish though – a lightbulb moment within a lightbulb moment, if you like – is discovering that there is a soft side to enough. A softness that restores my breathing, gives me hope and is walking me home. I am *enough* … I have *enough*.

These two small collections of words, six words, twenty letters and four dots, will be more healing for me than anything else could be. I am coming home.

Enough said?

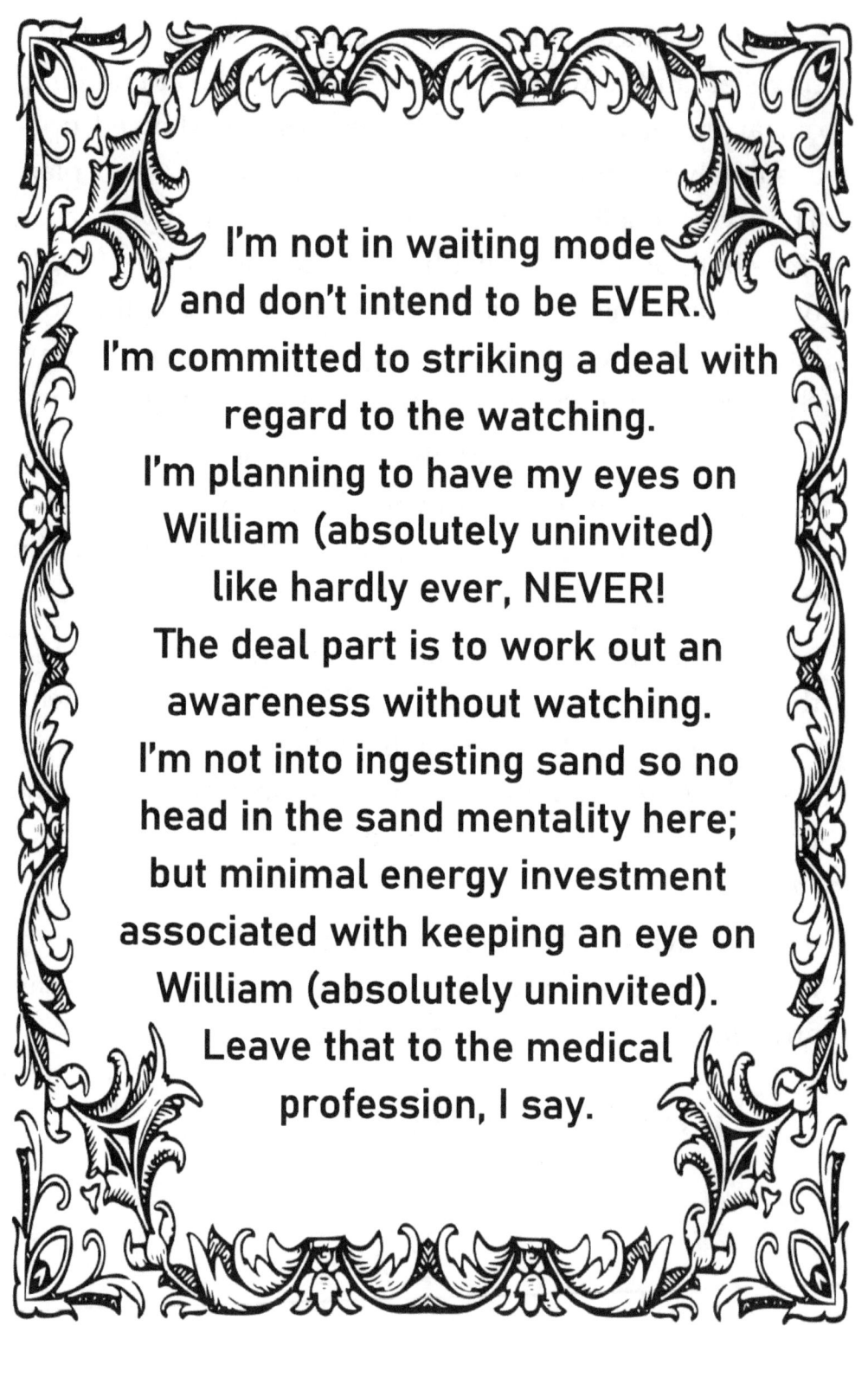

I'm not in waiting mode and don't intend to be EVER. I'm committed to striking a deal with regard to the watching. I'm planning to have my eyes on William (absolutely uninvited) like hardly ever, NEVER! The deal part is to work out an awareness without watching. I'm not into ingesting sand so no head in the sand mentality here; but minimal energy investment associated with keeping an eye on William (absolutely uninvited). Leave that to the medical profession, I say.

green eggs and ham

I am Sam. I am Sam. Sam I am.
That Sam-I-am, that Sam-I am!
I do not like that Sam-I-am.
Do you like green eggs and ham?

You've gotta love Dr Seuss!

Well, it's not quite green eggs and ham, however, my mind recited green eggs and ham most mornings as I whipped up my favourite cocktail. Who was I to question my mind?!

It's green, hold the eggs and ham! For eighteen months I started each day with green juice, pulp and all.

You may like them, you will see, you may like them in a tree …

Well, get comfortable, put your feet up and let me take you down the corridors of watch and wait … Watch! Wait! Intrigued? The best possible status for William (absolutely uninvited), so I've been told repeatedly and so I continue to debate, is to be on a watch and wait management program. Only there doesn't seem to be a program. The management part is largely down to me, which eventually dawned on me. I realised that I could take ownership of the management part and, in this moment, I took something of myself back.

What it really means is:

1. The rate at which the cancer cells are creating in the bone marrow, or the percentage of cells that are cancerous, based on a bone marrow sample, is low enough not to warrant treatment.
2. The measurement of the abnormal protein (IgM) in the blood does not warrant treatment;
3. The lymph nodes and spleen are not enlarged, indicating no tumours;
4. No haemorrhaging in the eyes, normal kidney function, no signs of damage to lungs and heart.

William (absolutely uninvited) has two heads ... A two-headed monster as it were! Off with its heads, I say!!!!

Head one: the abnormal protein, immunoglobulin (IgM) being transported around the body with the blood can deposit in the lymph nodes and/or spleen and cause tumours.

Head two: hyper-viscosity (thick, sticky blood caused by the extra abnormal protein) can cause a lack of oxygen supply to organs and eyes; chronic fatigue as the body works extra hard to circulate blood and oxygen; anaemia as B cell production may be diminished due to cancer cell production.

My conclusions:

1. I'm not in waiting mode and don't intend to be, *EVER*.

2. I'm committed to striking a deal with regard to the watching. I'm planning to have my eyes on William (absolutely uninvited), like hardly ever, NEVER! The deal part is to work out an awareness without watching. I'm not into ingesting sand so no head in sand mentality here; but minimal energy investment associated with keeping an eye on William (absolutely uninvited). Leave that to the medical profession, I say.

3. Stay healthy Sam-I-am … Health is a potent William (absolutely uninvited) repellent.

4. William (absolutely uninvited)! Your days are numbered!

The haematologist does the watching, and I'm guessing I do the waiting, or maybe that's down to William (absolutely uninvited)! Anyway, not important this waiting as I have other ideas and none of it even remotely resembles waiting!

Watch and wait. Who the fuck came up with that?

The green juice is gone, the cup is empty and all those superfoods are being absorbed into my body and promoting healthy cells and turning into energy …

Life, here I come!

Sometimes I am smiling
through tears and
dancing a slow rhythm
in my pyjamas;
there are days
when the mardi gras
just ain't going to happen,
no fruit bowl on my head,
no vibrant coloured twisting
skirt, but dance, I will.

show up! no matter what!

Every moment I feel blessed and grateful and I smile a lot.

Sometimes I am smiling through tears and dancing a slow rhythm in my pyjamas; there are days when the mardi gras just ain't going to happen, no fruit bowl on my head, no vibrant coloured twirling skirt, but dance, I will.

I will always dance and I will always smile.

I will show up, no matter what.

William (absolutely uninvited) you will not ever stop my dance and my song.

It's a fragile balance sometimes, and a frustrating appointment with my specialist can cause me to stumble.

Having a rare condition means that the medical profession, particularly in Bunbury it would seem, know very little to nothing about William (absolutely uninvited).

I saw the haematologist on the 16th of December 2014 for

the first time since receiving the diagnosis in a letter in the mail, in early July. Really, the alarm bells should have been going off then. Who the hell does that? Send a diagnosis of blood cancer by letter, in the mail and no appointment until six months later.

At the time, I was so very relieved that I didn't require chemotherapy that nothing else mattered. I was too tired from months of working and doing that I never thought about this before then.

I invited my children to come along to this particular appointment and meet the blood specialist who was overseeing the management of the very unwelcome William (absolutely uninvited). These two beautiful souls who had been on the South West Health Campus ride of your life with me for seven months … they had met Sam-I-am (and also don't like green eggs and ham) and had been terrified and vulnerable. My children had had the contents of their stomachs hit the roof of their mouths, cried with me, laughed with me and loved me unconditionally.

Having survived the war on William (absolutely uninvited) thus far, they strode into Raven's Cottage with me to meet the man who handed down a verdict that will forever ring out on the cobblestone path of their lives. *"You know your mother has something that will probably kill her?"*

"Did you slap her for getting those tattoos?" was this doctor's first question of me. He was referring to my beautiful Neesha. My beautiful daughter was twenty years old at the time. She has lived through many moments since then that no twenty-year-old should ever have to cope with. She had lain alongside me and cried with me when that was all that could get us through. Holding Neesha's hand, and her love, were defining moments that got me to my feet and dancing and smiling. Many times.

Then this medical professional (and I say this loosely) looked to Neesha and asked, "what will you do when you're in a nursing home with those tattoos and you're the odd one out?"

I was so disgusted and outraged I wanted to scream at him! Somehow I responded with "when Neesha is in a nursing home, the person with no tattoos will be the odd one out." I curiously observed my capacity to respond calmly with words when I am fucking furious inside.

I had a million questions to ask since diagnosis – and those were only the ones I knew about at the time!

I researched extensively between diagnosis and this appointment, compiling a resource folder on William (absolutely uninvited) from the International Waldenstrom's Macroglobulinemia Foundation website-based downloads (www.iwmf.com).

I joined a closed social media group, all members living with their own version of William (absolutely uninvited) or supporting someone who is.

I was slowly getting through the information and beginning to know my enemy, so to speak.

I was able to narrow my million questions to three for

this appointment. He dismissed them all without addressing a single one. With a "call me Monday for blood results", the doctor stood up and announced that the appointment was over. I paid $150 for blood tests and no answers. And tears came when I opened my eyes the next morning.

Frustration and despair.

Some days are spent undoing the impact of others.

I spend my energy releasing my anguish and letting go.

It's how it is.

No matter what, I turn up each day, I smile through the tears and I dance to the beat of the moment.

Incidentally, I decided to never see that haematologist again.

Unknowingly and uncannily, friends reached out and hugged me. They shared posts to my timeline on social media. I received an early morning phone call from my brother, an "I love you" from my son as he left for work and a phone call from a dear friend. The tears stopped, and the tempo became more upbeat, and I start to twirl.

I am enough.

I have enough.

Show up, no matter what!

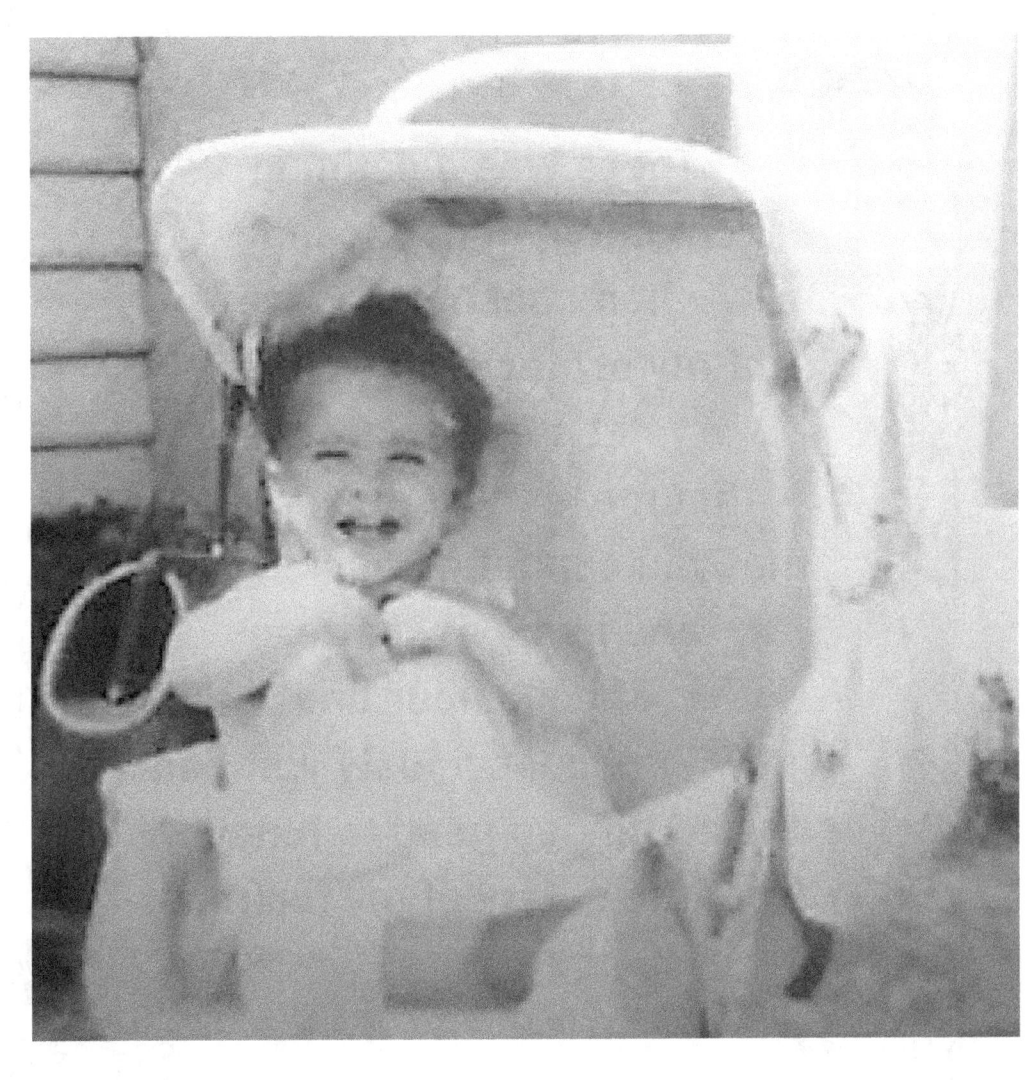

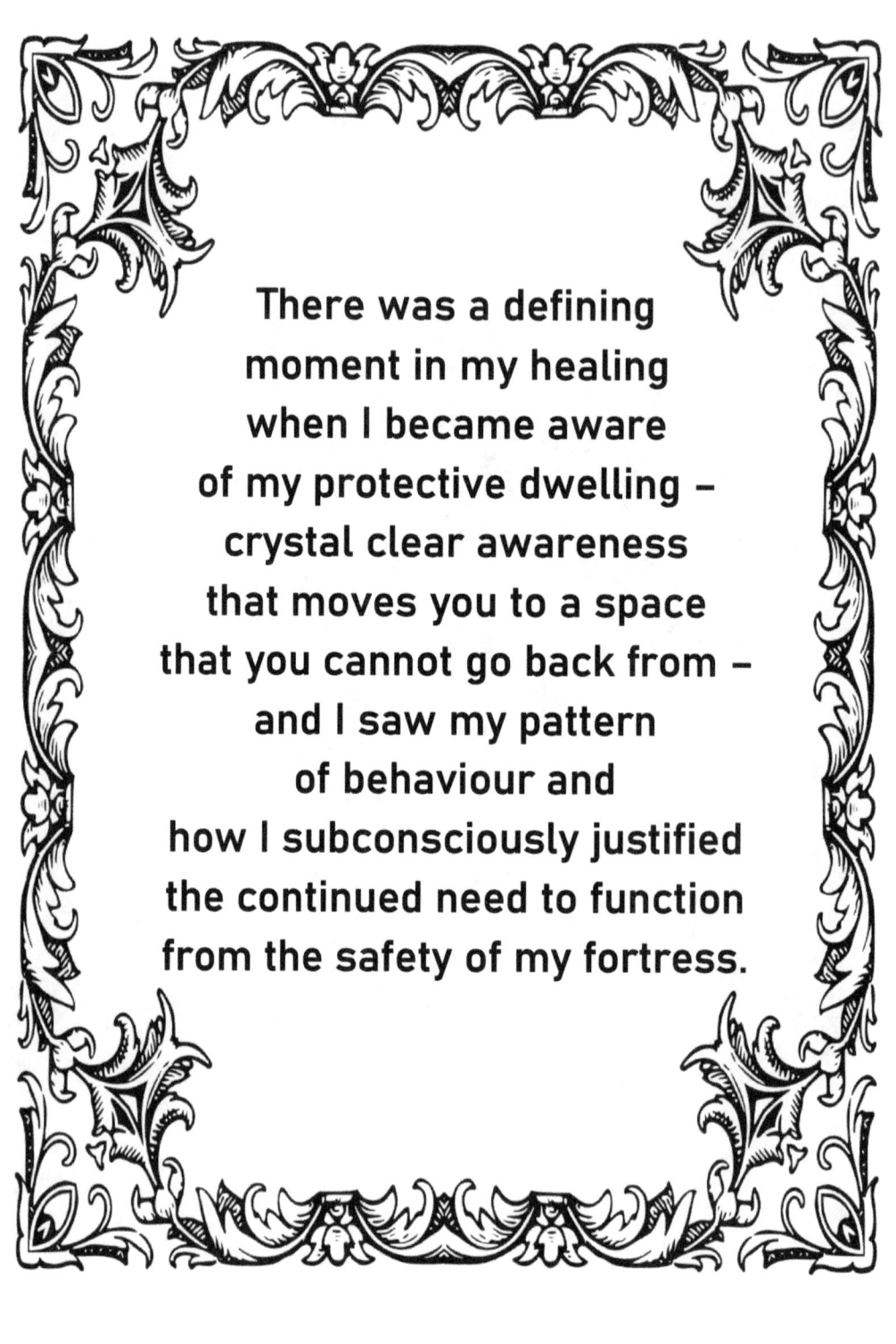

There was a defining
moment in my healing
when I became aware
of my protective dwelling –
crystal clear awareness
that moves you to a space
that you cannot go back from –
and I saw my pattern
of behaviour and
how I subconsciously justified
the continued need to function
from the safety of my fortress.

walking through vulnerability to courage

Impatient by nature (I'm an Aries woman!), I really wanted to fast-track to courage when confronted with William (absolutely uninvited).

I really have had to train my mind over the years to appreciate the detail level of things and the journey. I tend to make up my mind on matters and take the proverbial leap without a second thought. Then I start to ask AM I THERE YET?, because that's how I roll ... Decide and arrive, right?

Well, no. In reality, it's nothing like that, and it's been an interesting concept for me to grasp, this journey business. The universe has had to bring out the big guns for me to actually get this and metaphorically slap me in the face with it.

Okay, universe, I get it.

The plan to face this situation with strength and courage is a really good plan and one that will knock William on his uninvited arse.

What I didn't have a strategy for – and I really didn't see it coming – was that I would have to walk *through* my vulnerability on the road to finding the strength and courage – the inner gladiatrix.

I have always thought that to cry and feel sad is a weakness and not something that should be brought out and put publically on display. For most of my life, I have thought that one of the most hideous things I could ever do is to break down emotionally in the presence of another person.

I don't think there was anything I was more afraid of.

I'm afraid of many things, like spiders, sharks, angry men, violence, to name a few. Oh, and crying in public.

Very early in my life, I began construction of a fortress around my vulnerability. I was a small baby when I first feared for my safety, and the first stone was laid, the foundation of my fortress of self-protection.

I'm not aware of when my fortress reached lockup stage, or when I was handed the keys to my very first residence, but I know I don't have one memory of not being inside my fortress, protected from the world and whatever life would throw at me.

Until recently.

There was a defining moment in my healing when I became aware of my protective dwelling – crystal clear awareness that moves you to a space that you cannot go back from – and I saw my pattern of behaviour and how I subconsciously justified the continued need to function from the safety of my fortress.

I created and attracted conflict so I could validate a lifetime behind fortress walls.

Lower the drawbridge and let life in, she said.

In early 2015, many weeks were spent keeping that drawbridge down and inviting life in, warts and all.

Destruction of the fortress was not a difficult thing for me, it was a decision, and it was down in a cloud of dust, just like that. I totally accepted that this was what was right for me.

The challenge lay in the 'not picking up a brick' to lay a new foundation every time I felt unsafe.

It still is the challenge. And as the dust settled around the ruins of my fortress, I met my vulnerability. I was so frightened.

I had never seen anything so beautiful in my life.

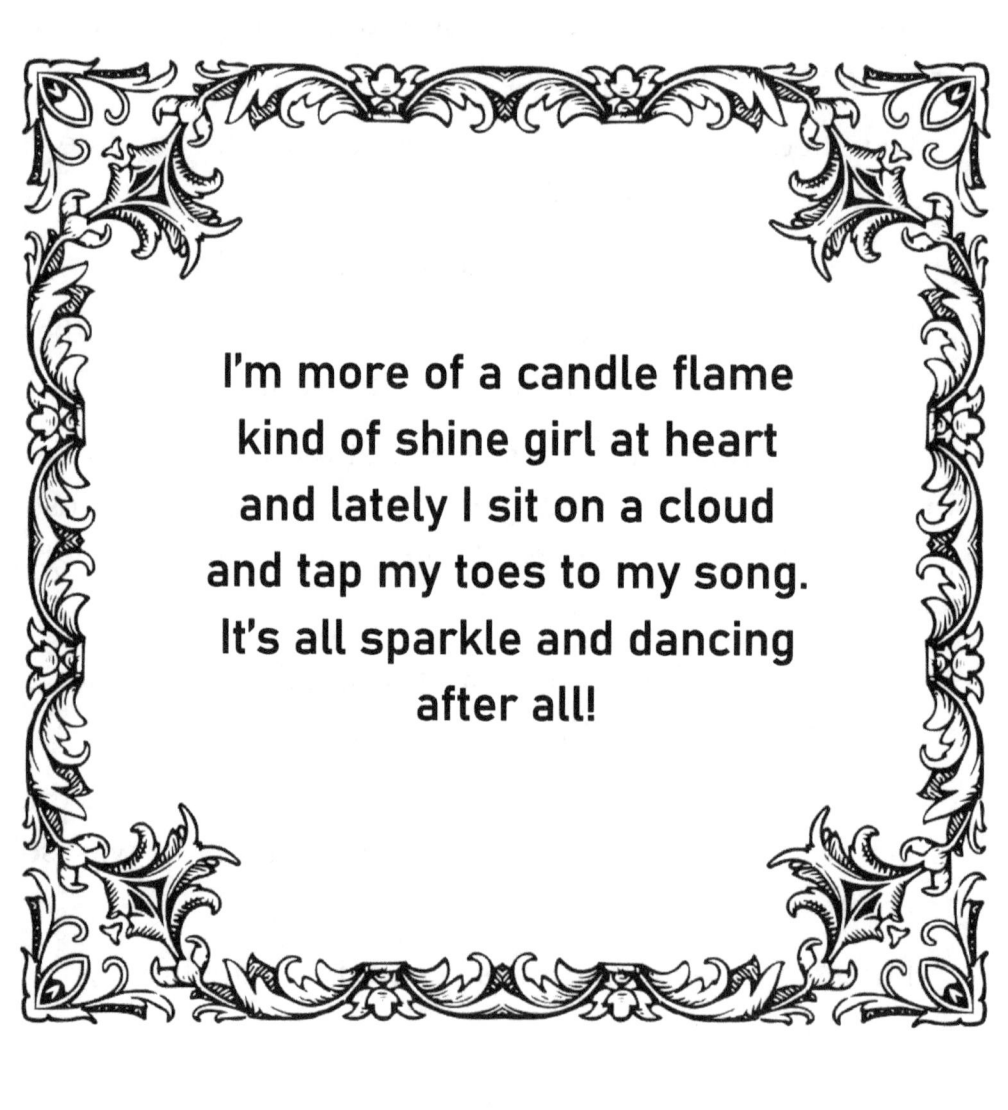

I'm more of a candle flame kind of shine girl at heart and lately I sit on a cloud and tap my toes to my song. It's all sparkle and dancing after all!

when i is replaced by we illness becomes wellness

Exhaustion is the topic of the day … the week … the month … many months and in fact, years now.

"I'm tired, but otherwise I'm well." That's usually how I respond when I'm asked how I am. It is true, but it so inadequately describes how I am.

Some days I feel like I'm bobbing around in a stormy ocean, like I've been here for a long time treading water. There are times I scrape the bottom of the dig-deep jar to stay afloat.

I am weary to the core and thoughts come and go. I observe them like visitors who come to the door – they knock a couple of times, call out and eventually leave, thinking I'm not home.

I have intent. I have wishes and ideas. These are the visitors who knock and I observe with no energy to do anything but watch them leave.

Thursday and Friday are the worst. It's like the energy jar empties by mid-week. I get by on love and a prayer from then until the weekend. This is not negativity, it is not depression. It is not feeling sorry for myself. This is chronic fatigue. It's exhaustion. Nothing more, nothing less. It is completely invisible. Chronic fatigue is a right bastard by any standard, and, just as uninvited as William.

Yet I continue to shine; more of a glow than a sparkle, but shine I do.

I'm more of a candle flame kind of shine girl at heart and lately I sit on a cloud and tap my toes to my song. It's all sparkle and dancing after all!

What can you do to help? Stay close, keep in touch, don't wait for me to ask for help, tell me jokes, believe in unicorns, have glitter on hand, wear a tiara, invite me to a tutu party in the morning. Just don't become invisible too!

When 'I' is replaced by 'we' 'illness' becomes 'wellness'.

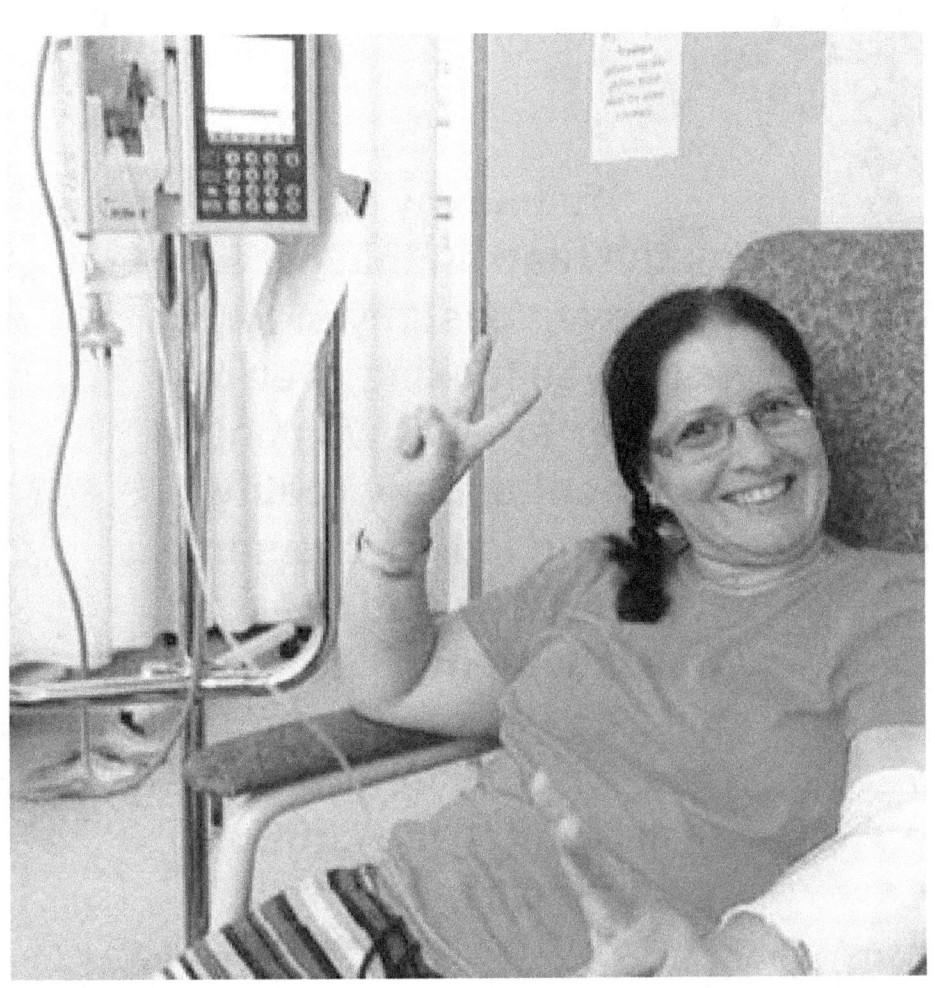

April, 2014

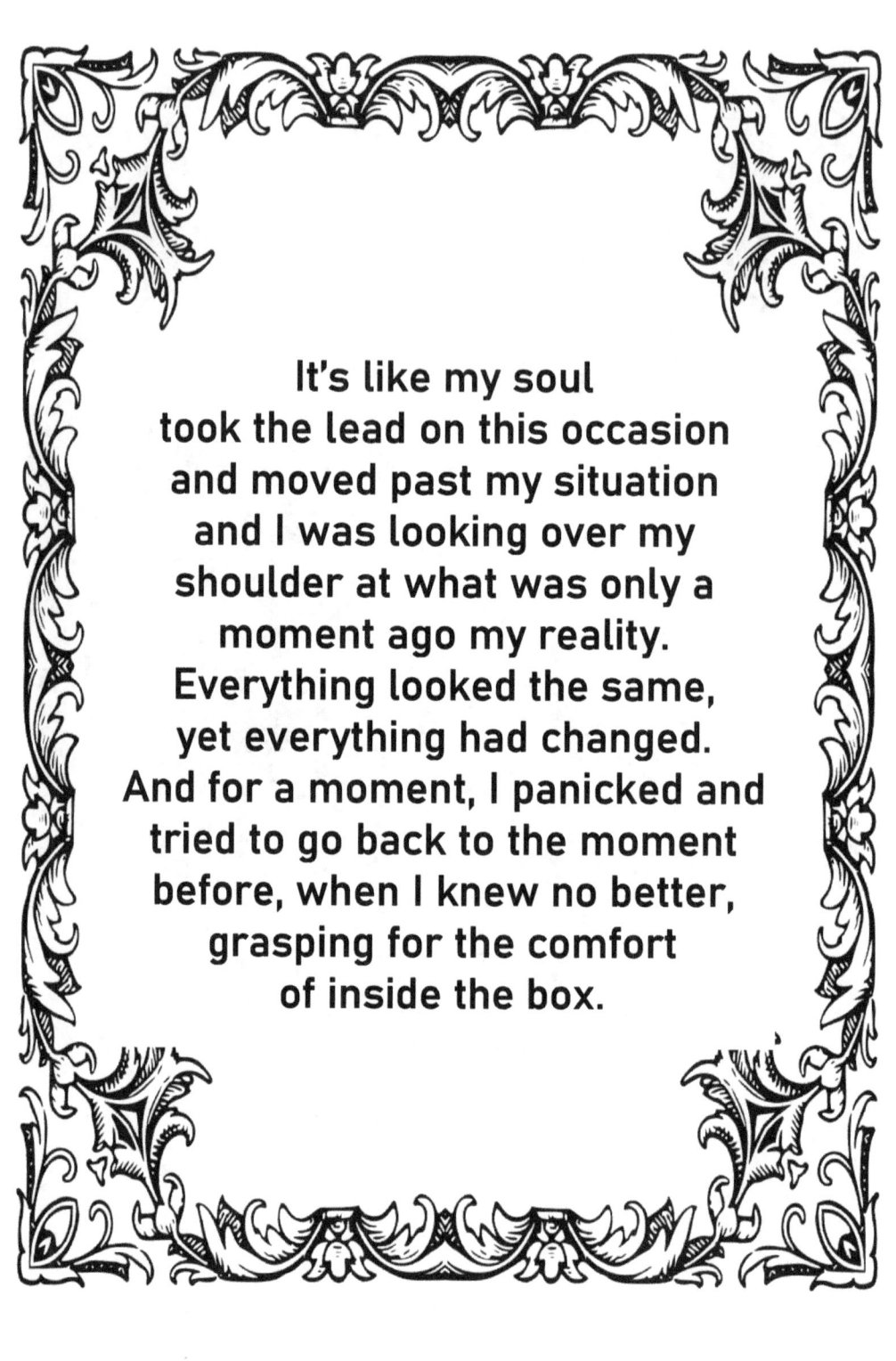

It's like my soul
took the lead on this occasion
and moved past my situation
and I was looking over my
shoulder at what was only a
moment ago my reality.
Everything looked the same,
yet everything had changed.
And for a moment, I panicked and
tried to go back to the moment
before, when I knew no better,
grasping for the comfort
of inside the box.

sweet surrender

I heard a whisper and realised it was my own voice. I found myself at the edge of my own existence, with all of my life experiences and all of my memories, all of who I am and who I have been, cloaked around me.

I've been struggling on this pathway, stumbling at times, not wanting to step on the cracks at other times, not wanting to step at all; paralysed by fear and uncertainty.

It's like my soul took the lead on this occasion and moved past my situation and I was looking over my shoulder at what was only a moment ago my reality. Everything looked the same, yet everything had changed. And for a moment, I panicked and tried to go back to the moment before, when I knew no better, grasping for the comfort of inside the box.

Surrender, let go, change is on the wind. Trust and flow from this, was the whisper that I heard.

I have no plan. I have truly let go and I have faith that I will have more than I need and my future will unfold and it will be beautiful.

I've spent most of my life worrying about my financial security. I continued to go to my job for eleven months after diagnosis, when I knew absolutely that this was not what was right for me. I continued to put my health second to my work. During this time, I had no energy for life outside of work and this was not a joyful way to live.

I told myself that my financial security was the most important thing, and I ignored the whispers of my soul, pushing on with the daily grind. Then the exhaustion came again and it's like we all sat at the table – fear, doubt, hope, faith, William (absolutely uninvited) and the voice of reason. It was noisy as fear and doubt stood on their chairs and beat their chests, protesting loudly, talking over the top of one another.

And out of this debate, I emerged, composed and calm, with faith and hope each holding my hand. I knew I was going to listen to the whisper of my soul and flow from that.

I surrendered. I stopped resisting.

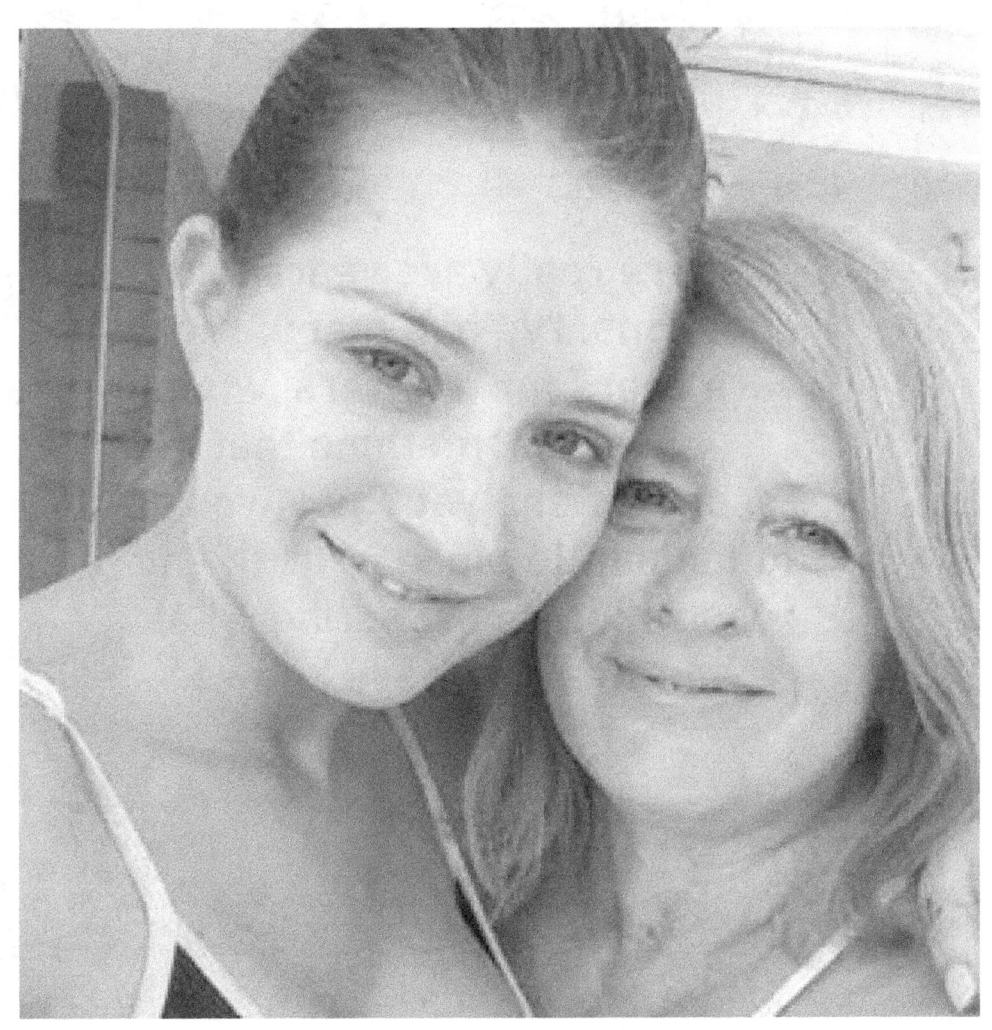

March, 2018

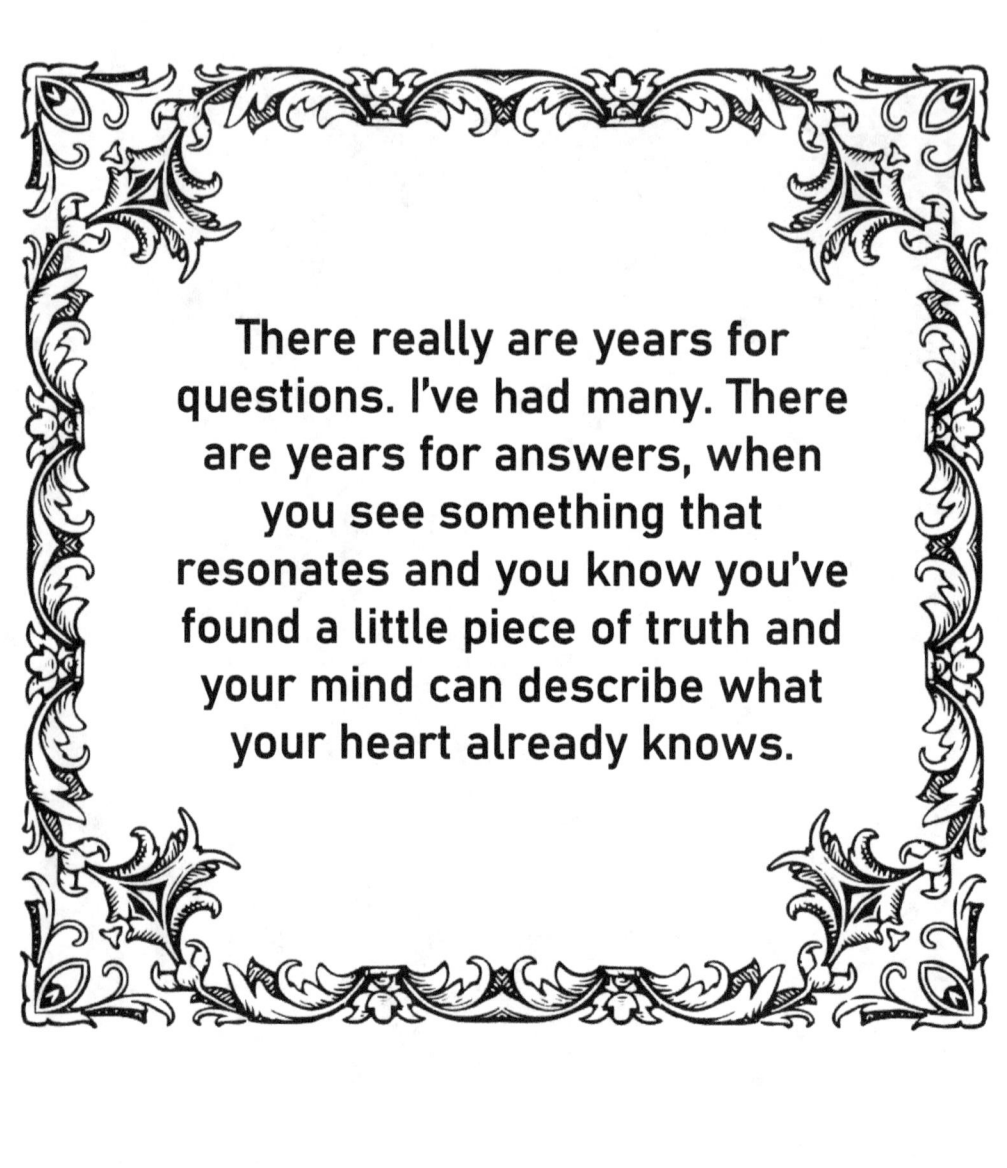

There really are years for questions. I've had many. There are years for answers, when you see something that resonates and you know you've found a little piece of truth and your mind can describe what your heart already knows.

let your heart walk you home

I've been questioning a lot lately; not feeling too comfortable in this space between where I was and where I will be. I've been making change by becoming the change I want – taking leaps of faith like I'm playing hopscotch.

There really are years in your life for questions. I've had many. There are years for answers, when you see something that resonates and you know you've found a little piece of truth and your mind can describe what your heart already knows.

When I collided head-on with William (absolutely uninvited) it's like I've passed through the wall of the train station on my way to Hogwarts. I've been really busy in my mind, trying to work out a plan to cope and live with William (absolutely uninvited). How to be what I needed to be, so my changes wouldn't affect those who counted on me not to change. It's no wonder I'm exhausted.

Smack! is the sound of the simplest truth hitting me in the face! Stop planning; that's not living, it's planning; stop trying to live with William (absolutely uninvited).

Just live.

I've made decisions that would have once been categorised as those of a madwoman. My inner critic has been having a field day with my mind. Yet, despite all the noise and chaos, I know that this was what I absolutely must do. I just didn't know why.

I have so many holes, so many heart bruises and life has been asking me to stop avoiding them. Life was asking me to no longer despise my holes and bruises and to no longer make them prettier than they are. To stop censoring myself, denying my heart and rejecting my gut. To stop and notice the bruising and the holes. To not seize the moment of truth but to recognise it and embrace it gently, like an old friend, to let my heart take me home. To recognise the beauty in the holes and the bruises and realise that these are the road on which I have walked my life and it is in the heart of this journey that my soul dwells.

Ssssshhhh … can I have some quiet, please. The time for questions has passed. Be still, be quiet and listen to the answers.

Freedom.

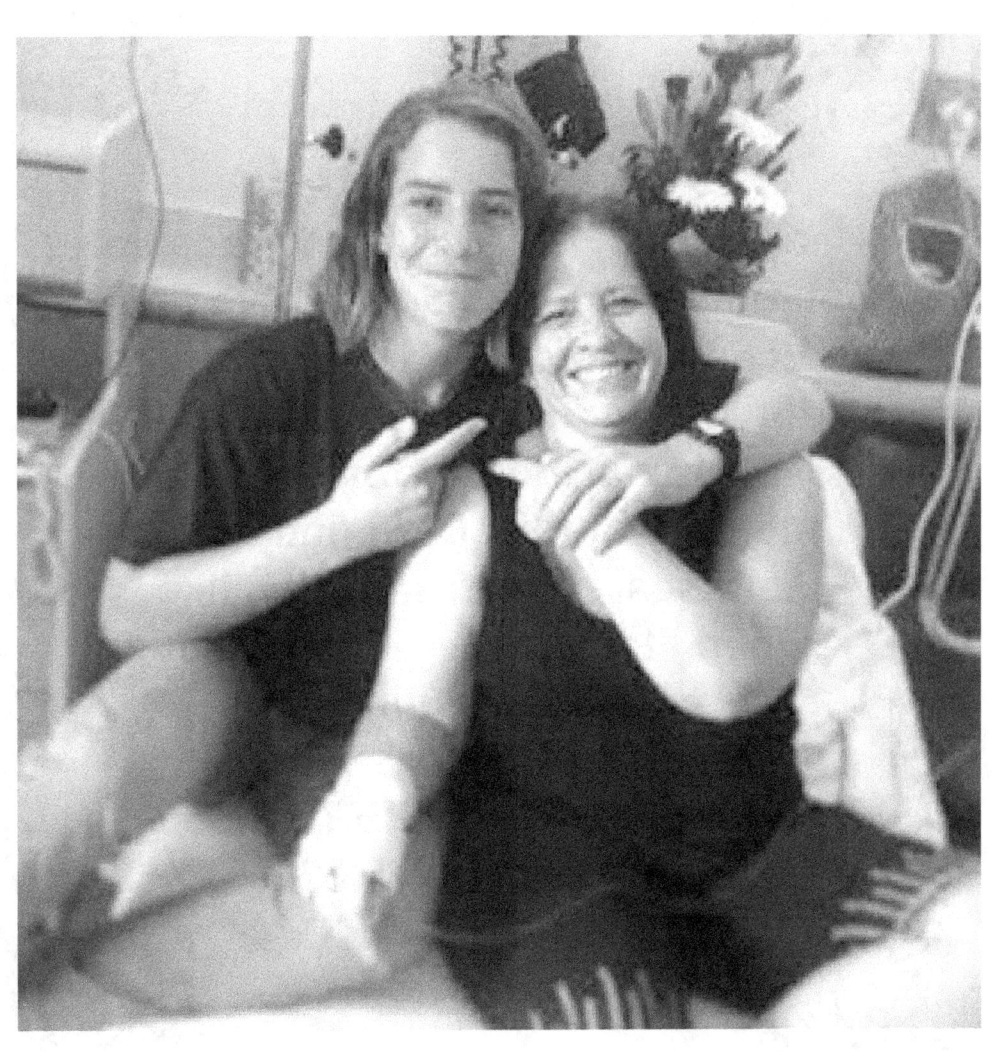

April, 2014

I am sitting here, trying to recall a time when I felt comfortable and accepting of my body. I'm opening the many doors and windows of my mind, looking for just one memory of this. I can find none. I am searching frantically, like when I lose something precious and I can't find it.
It's a desperation.
PLEASE LET THERE BE JUST ONE TIME?!

embodiment

Love your body, darling. It's been with you through it all. It's more faithful to you than anything else. It will love you unconditionally till its last breath. It will carry you for as long as it can. It will heal the cuts that come along as good as it can. It lets you know when you need to rest. It lets you know when you're getting too stressed. It tries to speak with you about a beauty you have that the world can't understand. It just has always and will ever always simply want to be your friend.

S.C. Lourie/butterfilesandpebbles

And there it is in black and white. The words that I stumbled upon just when I needed to. The words that sirened and screamed at me as this will be one of the biggest issues for me to overcome. I'm not even sure I can overcome the issues I have with how I feel about my body.

Mind, body and soul are what I am, and I'm doing okay with mind and soul. I see the body as the embodiment of my mind and soul, the tangible and visible form of me, so much more than a skeletal support structure.

embodiment (im/bodiment/) *noun*

tangible or visible form of an idea, quality, or feeling. The representation or expression of something in a tangible or visible form.

I am sitting here, trying to recall a time when I felt comfortable and accepting of my body. I'm opening the many doors and windows of my mind, looking for just one memory of this. I can find none. I am searching frantically, like when I lose something precious and I can't find it. It's a desperation. PLEASE LET THERE BE JUST ONE TIME?!

Okay, there is one environment in which I am unaware of my body image and as such, accepting my physical form – when I am alone. I have a lot of anxiety when I go outside my home, around the way I look. I have a constant battle between dressing in what I feel is comfortable and resonates and making sure that I hide my body.

I tend to go with what's comfortable and what resonates – colour, fabric and how it feels, but it's a real battle for me. I don't like to look in the mirror, but I absolutely must make sure my arse doesn't look too big in that. So it's a fleeting glance.

I won't swim in a social setting because I don't feel comfortable in bathers. I am embarrassed about cellulite and fat. I believe that one of the reasons I am on my own is because my body is not physically attractive. I don't have a fix for this issue. I can read all the positive words there are to be read, and that does not take away the fact that I feel shame, embarrassed and self-conscious about my body.

I don't want to fix my body, I want to accept myself totally no matter what I weigh; I want to accept the cellulite and fat. I want my body to be the tangible and visible representation of my mind and my soul.

I believe my diet and exercise needs must be focused on being healthy, not on having a toned and perfect body.

I have a very big mountain to climb here. Acknowledging this is hopefully the first step on the journey to reconciling my mind and my soul with my body.

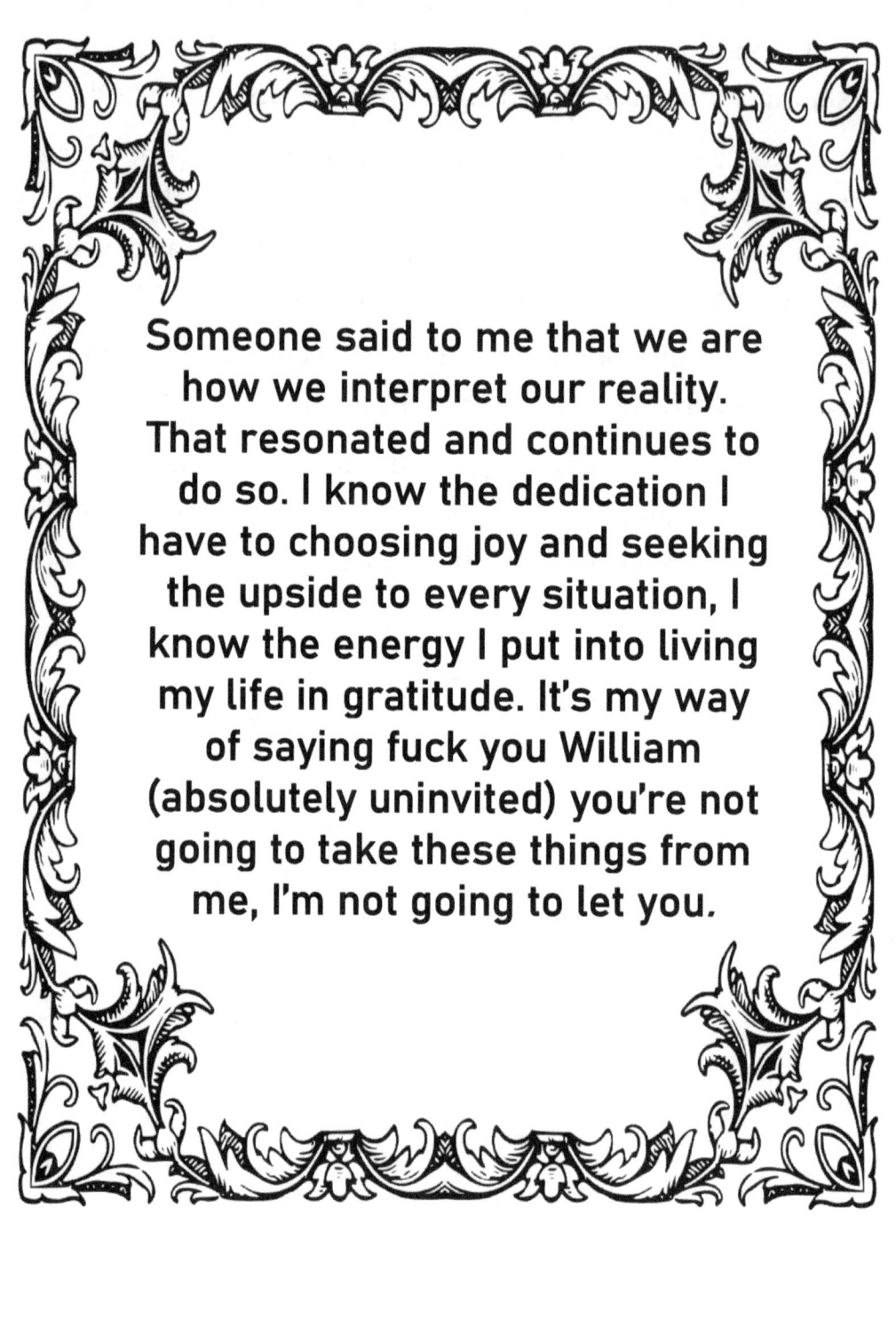

Someone said to me that we are how we interpret our reality. That resonated and continues to do so. I know the dedication I have to choosing joy and seeking the upside to every situation, I know the energy I put into living my life in gratitude. It's my way of saying fuck you William (absolutely uninvited) you're not going to take these things from me, I'm not going to let you.

my spiritual warrior

Anger is not only inevitable, but it is necessary. For in its place is indifference, the worst of all human qualities.

Anonymous

Sometimes I feel like the weather on a wild, stormy day is reflecting what's going on inside.

ANGRY.

Damn straight I'm angry.

I DESPISE and HATE cancer.

There, I said it out loud. Well, I bloody well shouted it with all my might. You bloody mongrel disease! Just get back on the flea-infested camel you rode in on and fuck off out of this life!!!!

Not only is it okay to be angry, but a very necessary part of my healing.

A friend and intuitive healer once said to me:

"Anger is healing too! It's as though our soul steps up and says, fuck off that which is causing us unnecessary pain. You are not worthy to be part of me. So go tell William to fuck off!

"Anger is like empowering yourself and your self-worth. It's a good healing tool. We love ourselves enough to be angry that something is trying to harm us. Takes us out of victim mode. So, strap on that armour, shield and sword and go kick its arse!"

God forbid that I ever become indifferent!

I know there is a lot to be thankful for, there is always someone worse off, blah blah … I know it, okay?! I don't ever lose sight of the things I have to be thankful for, the love I have for my children, beauty everywhere and life's miracles.

Sparkles and unicorns, tutus and tiaras are permanent fixtures in my life, not just something I bring out to cheer myself up.

I'm angry.

I haven't lost sight of everything else.

Someone said to me that we are how we interpret our reality. That resonated and continues to do so. I know the dedication I have to choosing joy and seeking the upside to every situation; I know the energy I put into living my life in gratitude. It's my way of saying fuck you William (absolutely uninvited)! You are not going to take these things from me. I'm not going to let you.

Am I grateful for the love and kindness I have had showered upon me these past four years?

You bet!

Do I miss the toilet seat left up level of life challenges?

Not for a minute!

Would I give everything to be cured of cancer and for the world to be cancer free?

Damn straight.

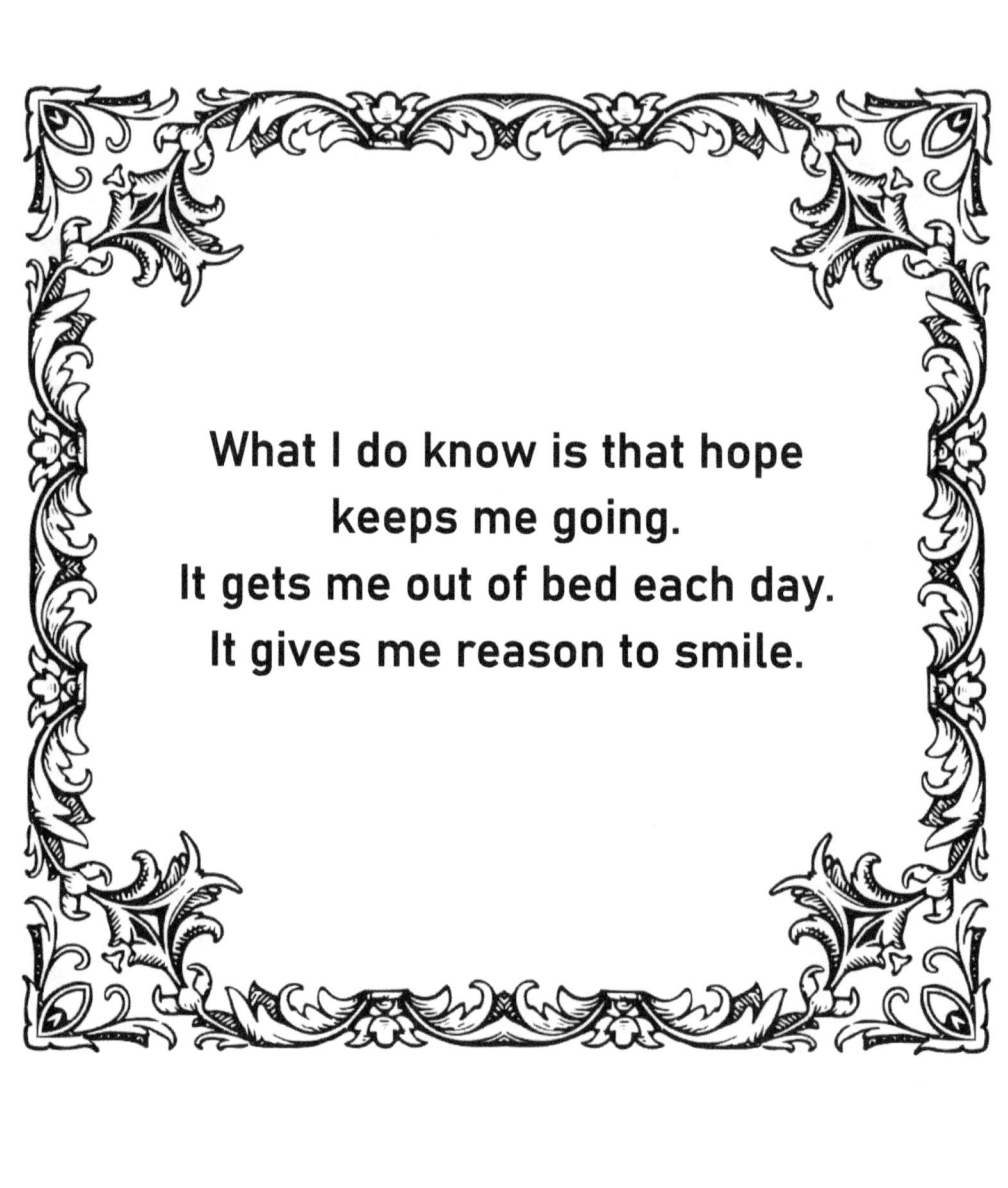

What I do know is that hope keeps me going.
It gets me out of bed each day.
It gives me reason to smile.

hope the little voice that whispers maybe

I think about hope. A lot. What is hope? Is it a wish? I've thought about the things I hoped for throughout my life.

I hoped my netball team would win and that I'd get to play the whole game.

I hoped I would get a kitten for my birthday.

I hoped I would pass my driving test.

I hoped I would pass exams.

I hoped to travel.

I hoped my child would be born healthy. I also prayed for this.

Is hope a prayer?

I hoped I got the job, I liked the job, got a pay rise; that I didn't miss the bus.

Fifty-five-year-old me hopes that I wake up each day with good health and joy in my heart.

I hope that my children are happy and healthy and the same for my family and friends.

I hope for world peace.

I hope for an end to poverty, famine and disease.

I hope that cancer is only a star sign.

Is hope the soft side of worry? Is hope what motivates?

I've looked at some of the definitions and quotes about hope.

> hope *noun*
> 1. a feeling of expectation and desire for a particular thing to happen.
> 2. archaic - a feeling of trust.

> Hope is being able to see that there is light despite all of the darkness.
>
> *Desmond Tutu*

> Hope is a waking dream.
>
> *Aristotle*

> Hope is patience with the lamp lit.
>
> *Tertullian*

> Hope is the pillar that holds up the world. Hope is the dream of a waking man.
>
> *Pliny the Elder*

> Hope is important because it can make the present moment less difficult to bear. If we believe that tomorrow will be better, we can bear hardship today.
>
> *Thich Nhat Hanh*

> My favourite: Hope is the thing with feathers that perches in the soul – and sings the tunes without the words – and never stops at all.
>
> *Emily Dickinson*

I've hoped for many things and sometimes my hopes come through.

Both of my children were born beautiful, healthy babies.

I got to go on an amazing trip to Paris for my 50th birthday celebrations.

Sometimes hope comes crashing down.

I hoped that I would not have cancer.

I hope with each blood test that I no longer have cancer.

There is a deep connection to vulnerability and courage when we have hope.

What I do know is that hope keeps me going. It gets me out of bed each day. It gives me reason to smile.

Hope is like the canvas on which life's miracles appear.

It's the flower that grows against all odds.

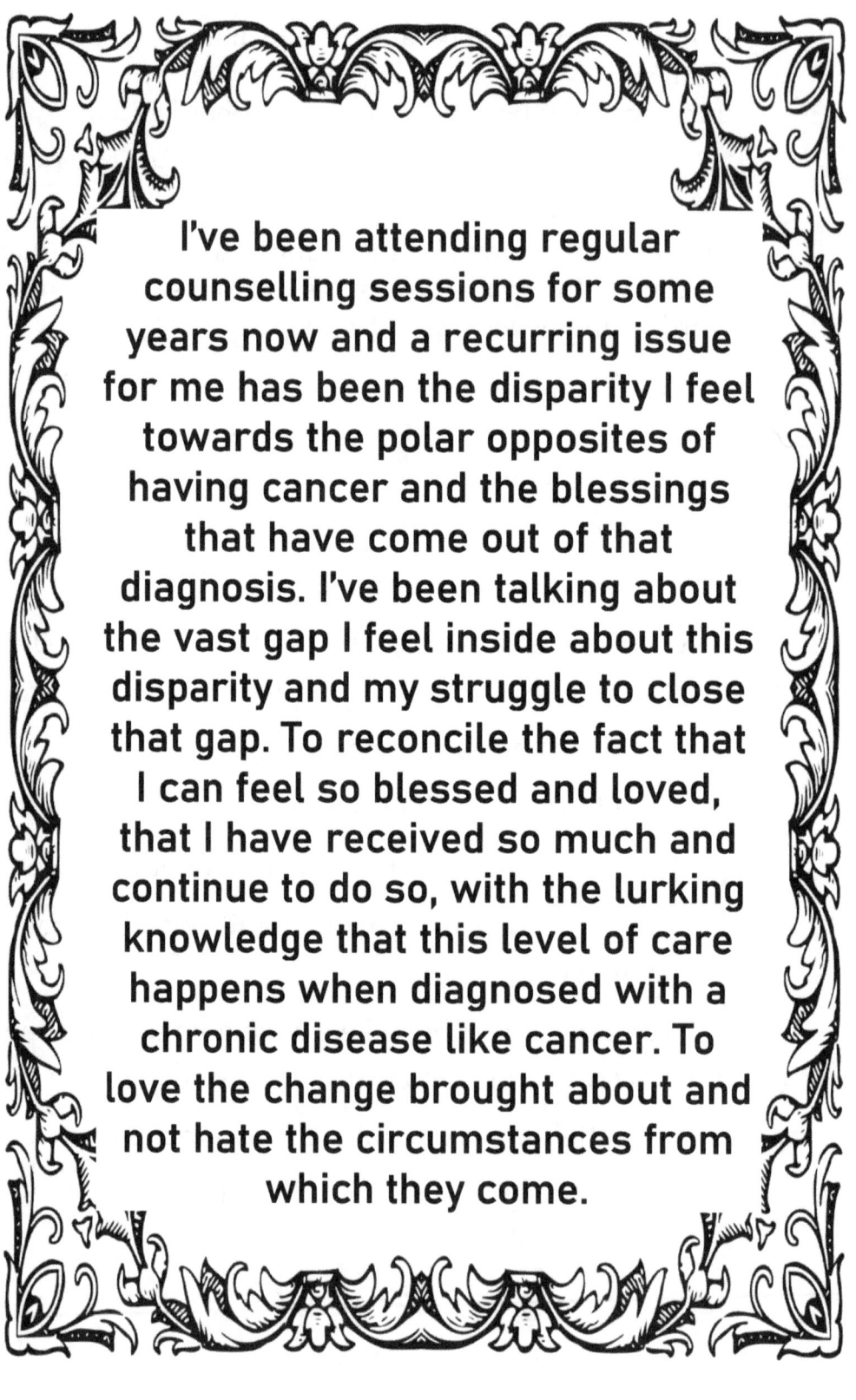

I've been attending regular counselling sessions for some years now and a recurring issue for me has been the disparity I feel towards the polar opposites of having cancer and the blessings that have come out of that diagnosis. I've been talking about the vast gap I feel inside about this disparity and my struggle to close that gap. To reconcile the fact that I can feel so blessed and loved, that I have received so much and continue to do so, with the lurking knowledge that this level of care happens when diagnosed with a chronic disease like cancer. To love the change brought about and not hate the circumstances from which they come.

is that joy i see up ahead?

I've read the book *The Invitation* by Oriah Mountain Dreamer. I was given the verses of *The Invitation* by a dear friend who warms my heart and always connects me to joy deep in my belly.

The language, the message in each of these verses, flow like honey over my soul. This stuff really speaks to me and resonates like an echo.

I was content to cherish the verses forever and read them until my fingers left marks on the laminate that covers the paper on which the words glisten.

I came across the book - I didn't even know there was a book! - in the conservative library at Solaris Cancer Care. It beckoned me! And I ordered the book on Amazon from a second-hand book shop in America and I now have my own copy.

My giddy aunt!!! I am poring over the pages, just a couple each day and my soul is drinking from this river indeed!

Then I read about the joy - the moments of impossible joy and realised how beautiful my life really is and the abundance of joy that I have felt, albeit not always recognised.

This chapter talks about joy in both the ordinary everyday moments and also in the extraordinary moments found in the experience of connection. This connection is the place where each of us receives the sense that we belong.

Oriah talks of emerging from the direct experience of who she is and how she laughed at the realisation that her worries about the future and hurts about the past, in that moment, were very small; how she knew in that moment that real joy does not deny what is hard in our lives.

I knew that I have been choosing joy around only the parts of my life that are not hard.

Joy - real joy - does not deny what is hard in my life.

I've been attending regular counselling sessions for some years now. A recurring issue for me has been the disparity I feel towards the polar opposites of having cancer and the blessings that have come out of that diagnosis. I've been talking about the vast gap I feel inside about this disparity and my struggle to close that gap. To reconcile the fact that I can feel so blessed and loved, that I have received so much (and continue to do so) with the lurking knowledge that this level of care happens only when diagnosed with a chronic disease like cancer. To love the change brought about and not hate the circumstances from which they come.

Then I read: Joy - real joy - does not deny what is hard in our lives. And that gap of disparity became smaller.

I read about resisting voices - both inner and outer - that tell me I must choose between joys, must pick a set of joys that fits a lifestyle.

Being with joy means being willing to expand - to hold it all – not to limit joy to fit an outcome. It means having joy about what I do well and about what I do badly.

It's about choosing not to participate, even by remaining silent, in another person's efforts to diminish the enormity in my life.

It's about not writing the ending at the beginning, complete with all the identifiable worst possible scenarios, to somehow avoid disappointment along the way.

It's about inviting joy into this moment whether it is a great moment or a not so great moment.

It's about revelling in the gardens, the beautiful French lights, the vitality of the Champs élysées on my way to the Arc de Triumph!

That gap of disparity grows smaller yet again. Oh, how joyful I am right now.

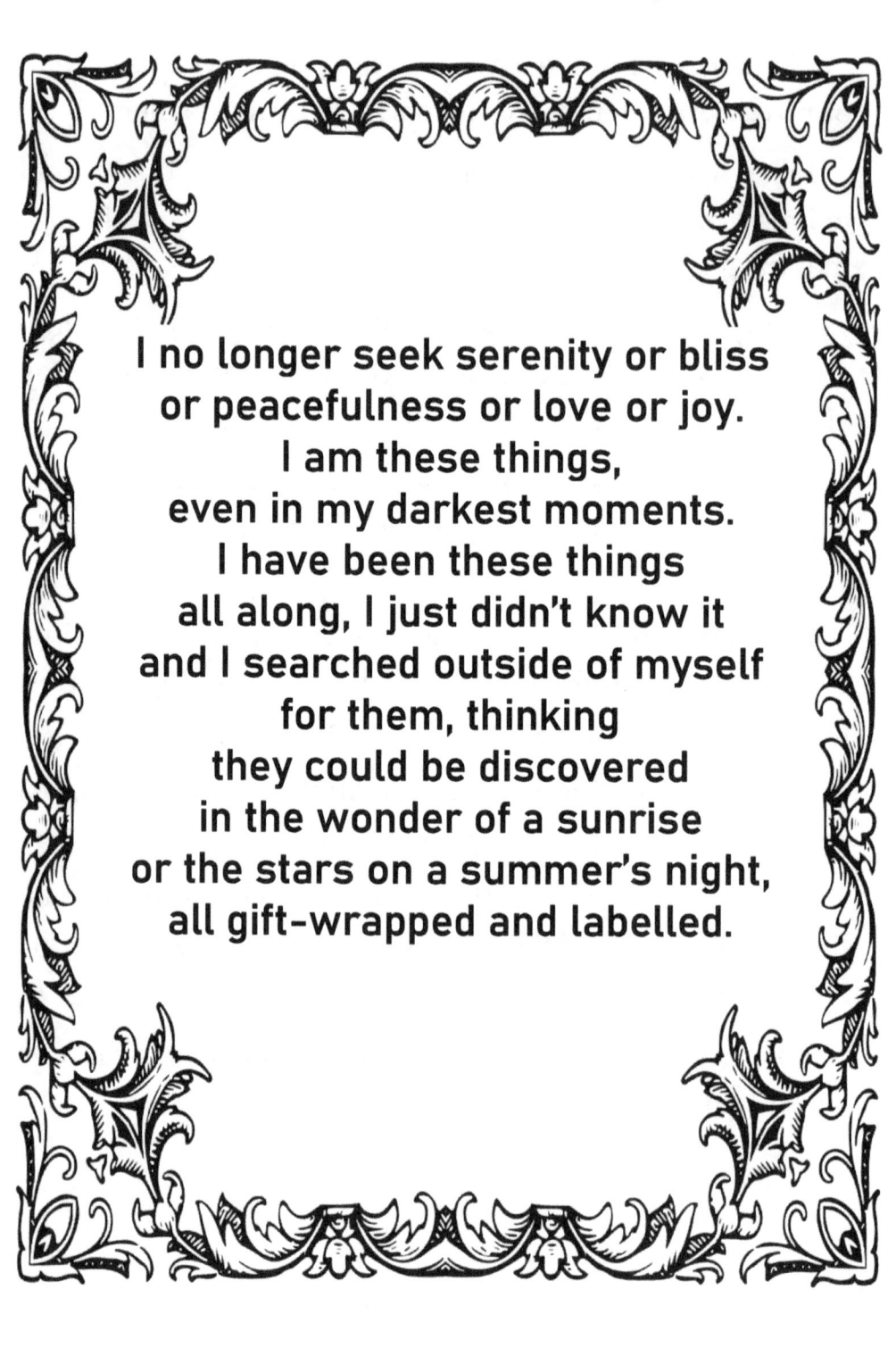

I no longer seek serenity or bliss
or peacefulness or love or joy.
I am these things,
even in my darkest moments.
I have been these things
all along, I just didn't know it
and I searched outside of myself
for them, thinking
they could be discovered
in the wonder of a sunrise
or the stars on a summer's night,
all gift-wrapped and labelled.

heart of the matter or matter of the heart?

To get to the heart of the matter, it really is necessary to see a situation for what it really is, warts and all, to know fully what one is dealing with so you can even remotely hope to work out how to cope; how to move forward.

The fundamental shortfall I have found with every self-help book and positive quote is that these fail to touch on the problem at hand. They fail to talk about the emotions and issues that send me looking, in desperation, for something to help me through. They have created this illusion that, if I affirm and believe life will be perfect and all, the hard-stuff struggles will go away. Imagine my complete and utter gobsmackedness after years of affirmations and believing that nothing but 'awesome' was going to come my way, when along came William (absolutely uninvited) and challenged these concepts and my own existence to its very core.

I want to express the gazillion emotions I have felt since William plonked himself unceremoniously and absolutely uninvited into my life. I want to talk about the very real issues that have presented to me in the past six years.

anxiety

Living with an incurable and rare blood cancer, on a watch-and-wait status, almost demands anxiety. The level of stress on my mind is layered and tiered and varies all of the time. I wonder who came up with such a thoughtless label – Watch and Wait: a label to describe the point of cancer where you do not require treatment but must be monitored regularly (to check that you haven't reached the point of needing treatment) … with the wait bit suggesting it's only a matter of time before treatment will be needed. Then throw in the bit about this being such a rare cancer that my doctor has never had a patient with Waldenstrom's Macroglobulinaemia before me. Add to that there is no specialist in Bunbury that knows and understands Waldenstrom's Macroglobulinaemia in such a way that they can actually answer my questions and offer support or management on a competent level.

Through the chaos of the initial diagnosis of cancer (but not the specific type), bone marrow biopsy, waiting for results, specific diagnosis and six-monthly tests with a one week wait for results, anxiety peaks. As I struggle with the awareness that my brain function, memory and mental and physical fatigue is an ongoing problem, I worry about my future and what will become of me.

assistance at home

I endured the process of arranging assistance with the home tasks that I can no longer manage. This was a four-tiered assessment process whereby you are questioned repeatedly about what you can and cannot do for yourself, a process which emphasises that you can no longer manage the things that you used to manage without thought. A process that tugs at the very core of hopelessness, with my anxiety going up and down wildly. Nevertheless, I am extremely grateful for fortnightly domestic assistance and monthly lawn mowing!

welfare

Being rejected for a disability support pension by Centrelink over three and a half years and three applications (because I was only assessed at 10/20 points of disability and therefore not eligible) triggered heightened anxiety and anger and frustration. Trying to survive on the Newstart payment of $577.50 a fortnight ($288.75 per week) takes its toll. I was assessed as unable to work, but for some reason, was not assessed as worthy of a disability support pension. And, while I am pleased to acknowledge that on appeal, my third application for disability support pension was successful (and I am now receiving the welfare payment that is right for me) I know there are many people living with disability who cannot access the right payment for them and are overwhelmed by the system.

foodbank

Shopping for food each week at Foodbank has opened my eyes to a layer of poverty that never in my wildest dreams could I have imagined. I have discovered that Foodbank is not this amazing supermarket designed for those less fortunate. I thought it might be like a Coles or Woolworths subsidised for the poor. It is not.

What is on offer is basically whatever is donated and in no way gravitates around the concepts of nutrition and/or health, **in no way whatsoever**. In the three years since I have been able to access Foodbank, the most available food types have been bread rolls, sticky buns and potato crisps with a variety of fruit and vegetables consisting mainly of overripe seasonal fruit and vegetables – sometimes with mould. On occasion, there are only green potatoes and onions available. However, the rules are that, to access Foodbank, each patron must purchase five kilos of fruit and vegetables. Sadly, the reality is that more often than not five kilos is not available.

At Foodbank, there are three aisles of packaged food, most of which is out of date – regularly more than 12 months out of date. Often, but not always, there is a small amount of meat. Occasionally, there is milk. There are no toiletries, toilet paper, cleaning products, tissues, laundry powder or liquid, dishwashing liquids, none of the non-food things you need to have.

It is not possible to eat my way to health from the shelves at Foodbank.

I want to acknowledge that I have felt myself at the very edge of my coping, many times. I have grasped for anything that will keep me from falling into a chasm of despair and hopelessness.

I have examined my own vulnerability and sought courage. I have recognised hope; and faith; and shame. I have looked into my own soul many times.

I have discovered a peacefulness and a wondrousness that can only be discovered from living at the very edge of my own existence.

I no longer seek serenity or bliss or peacefulness or love or joy. I am all of these things, even in my darkest moments. I have been these things all along, I just didn't know it. I searched outside of myself for them, thinking they could be discovered in the wonder of a sunrise or the stars on a summer's night, all gift-wrapped and labelled.

I have noticed the blissful silence that resonates answers to questions that hadn't occurred to me yet, at the times when I felt so alone and unsupported that it was just me and the universe in the room.

I have known the feeling of humanity like a gentle stroke on my skin when I had all but ran out of hope. When I sat curled tightly in the corner with the lights out and wishing that the torment would end. Then, unexpectedly, a friend knocked on my door with a meal and a message that I inspire them.

I have learned to receive, out of pure need, like I have never before received, nor imagined what it felt like on this level. When I know that I have nothing to give in return, other than absolute conviction to get up each day and fight this disease and to not give in to hopelessness and despair.

Healing has come my way, services that offer support, gifts, hugs and such love as I have ever known or knew existed. I speak to the universe all the time and I invite abundance and healing and protection for the essence and hearts of my children, who have their own difficult struggle with this cancer journey. I can't speak of their journey here as it is not my journey, but theirs and theirs alone to tell. Other than to say, that I am deeper than I ever thought possible through digging for courage and resolve, time and time again and I am capable of enduring the unimaginable because **I will not give up and I will not let my children slip through the ragged open chasms of this disease.**

I meditate with such hope and intent, seeking healing and checking out of this tough existence just for a while. Putting down the load and the thoughts and freeing my mind – like opening the window and letting in the sunlight and a gentle summer's breeze.

I have Reiki on a regular basis, to help keep my chakras aligned and to assist with healing.

I have Reflexology on a regular basis, to help with healing my body, through my feet.

I go to Harp Therapy religiously. I know, unequivocally, that this resets me, mind, body and spirit. I need this like I do oxygen.

I have counselling on a regular basis. In these moments, I see how far I've come and purge as much one can in an allocated hour.

I go to yoga and tai chi weekly.

I green juiced every day for 18 months, joyfully sourcing many of the ingredients from my beloved vegetable garden at the side of my house.

I take health supplements each day because I believe these help to boost my immune system, support healthy cell development and in part contribute to the energy that gets me out of bed every day and into my life.

I journal gratitude every other day.

I burn anger by writing it down and setting it alight, initially daily, now as required.

I write songs.

I play my Hapi Drum and my guitar.

I laugh fully, to the stage of happy tears and sore facedness and almost peeing myself a little. Unadulterated belly laughs!

I talk to the universe and I pray, like you wouldn't believe.

I see the miracles of life all around me, every minute of every day.

I have many, many moments of pure joy.

I scream and I cry… lots.

I read positive quotes.

I write "shinetime" quotes on my facebook page. These are usually designed around what I need to remind myself of at that time.

I blog.

I podcast.

I write books.

I spend every minute of every day making sure that I am okay in a situation that is not okay. This does not equate to having a negative mindset, it does not allude to me being a victim; I am a survivor.

What I have learned along this journey is that to fight this fight, I must know myself and fully accept my situation – a good deal of my emotional pain throughout my life has flowed from my inability to accept the situation at the time.

I have learned that to be courageous, I must first be vulnerable. This is not just a 10-letter word to be skipped over. No, sir! This means that I must open myself up, my heart in particular. Open heartedness means that I feel absolutely everything. Always. I feel the despair, the sadness, the frustration, the anger and the fear. The joy, love, hope and faith as well.

Healing and being positive is not about dismissing the things that make us feel sadness, anger and fear. Living authentically requires that we accept ourselves fully. Coping with life in a positive way, and authentically, means embracing all emotions. Understanding ourselves fully means sitting these dark emotions on our knee and having a conversation with that part of who we are; getting to know it, understand it and accept it. To love ourselves fully.

Trusting that everything is going to be okay if it's not okay at the time - accepting that you don't need to know the how or the why or the when. Knowing that every moment is unique in its flash of existence and a necessary part of your journey, even if it feels dreadful.

You see, matters of the heart really do require that we get to the heart of the matter. Life isn't some romantic fantasy where we get to create a knight in shining armour on a magnificent white unicorn to scoop us up behind them and ride off into the sparkles and sunset to live happily ever after – those are the fantasies that help us to cope with life. Life is about learning to love ourselves fully.

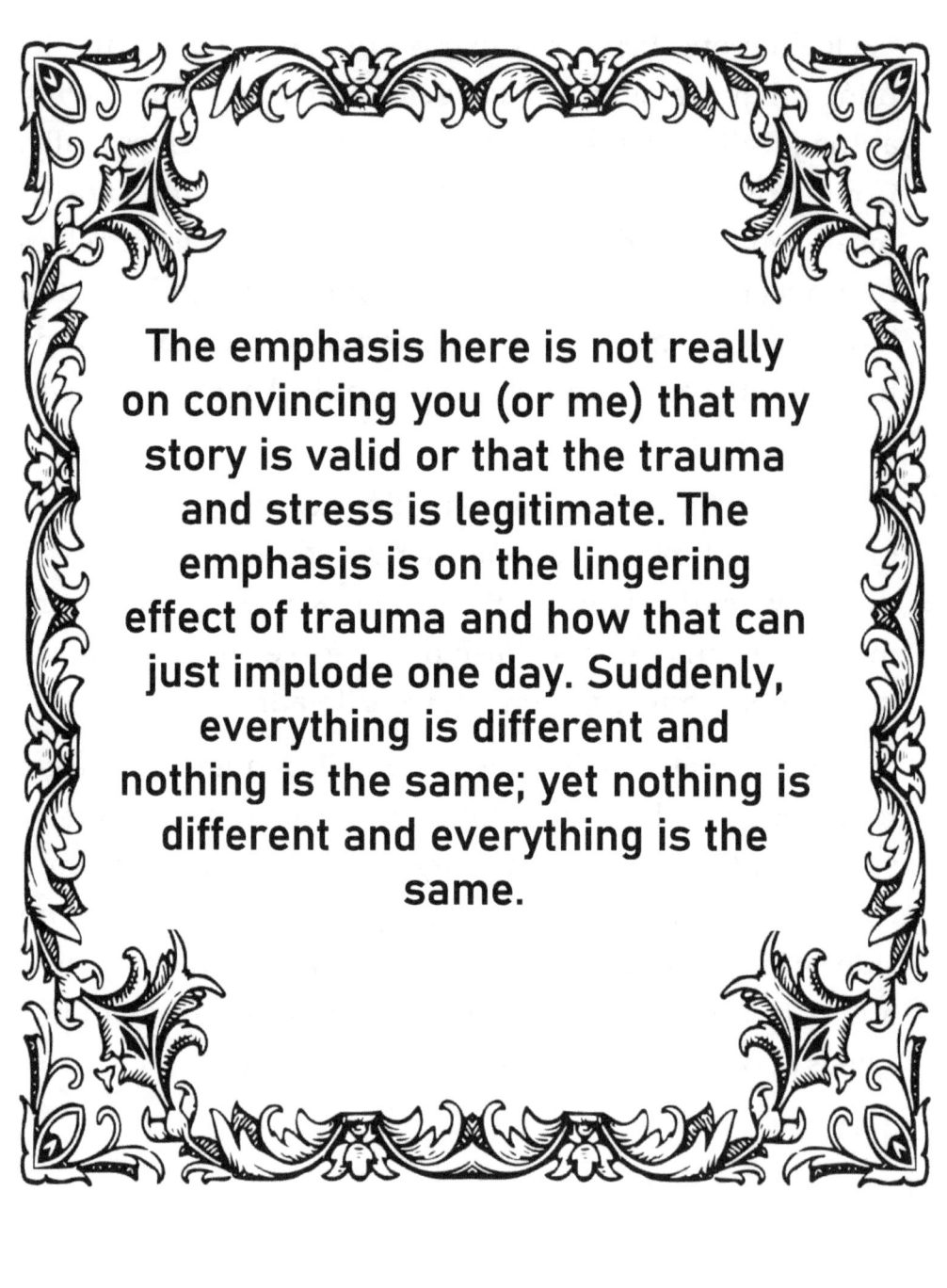

The emphasis here is not really on convincing you (or me) that my story is valid or that the trauma and stress is legitimate. The emphasis is on the lingering effect of trauma and how that can just implode one day. Suddenly, everything is different and nothing is the same; yet nothing is different and everything is the same.

i've been living in a war zone where there is no war

By my third appointment with a new therapist, I knew with certainty and truth that I had PTSD.

Only then was I able to begin to understand what had happened to my mind and psyche. And it was a very bare understanding; one that gave me hope that I was not going completely insane.

I need to be honest here about what I was feeling. To do this, I will touch on some things that I have been through that are so very personal to me, things I can only whisper because I carry such emotional pain around them. It's *my* stuff, that I keep closed in *my* heart and body, so please, if you're reading this, know that I am showing you a very vulnerable part of myself and treat it with respect.

On the 21st of March 2014, William (absolutely uninvited) arrived in my life, only I didn't really know it was him until the 26th of June 2014. Since then I have endured chronic fatigue and high anxiety while taking every step possible to improve my physical health and pleading with the universe to take William (absolutely uninvited) away just as magically as he had appeared and to keep myself on the right side of insane.

I could tell you the light and fluffy version of this existence – which is probably what you would like to hear – I've counted my blessings for every day that I've been here since and I am joyful every day because I choose this. I stay positive every moment, knowing God would never give me anything I couldn't handle.

But, I'm not going to do that.

I lived that existence for many, many years when my life was so damned hard. Believing that I could transform the hardships by sheer choice of thought and determination and while I didn't struggle with my mind due to this self-brainwashing, I didn't attract the life I so much wanted. I attracted William (absolutely uninvited).

It's been 2,530 days since William arrived amid a bursitis staph infection, chronic anaemia and high blood pressure. 2,530 days of feeling so tired that it's a struggle to function. I feel every bit of that struggle every minute of every day. I am constantly pushing myself to get up and do, partly for the fear that if I don't, I will stop existing and partly because

I am rebelling with all my might. 2,530 days of brain fog, losing my words mid-sentence (I became very adept at covering this), not remembering a movie I've watched, a conversation I've had; that I asked that very question two minutes ago; or whether I brushed my teeth or washed my face; if I locked the house before I left; wondering where I am going when I find myself driving somewhere and forget where that is.

I have many days where I decide to do something, go somewhere and turn around and come home before I get there; fighting a panic attack and spending hours trying to ground myself again. Then there are days when I am able to push through the fear and refuse to give in to it; still spending hours recovering from the adrenal fatigue and energy drain that this takes.

2,530 days of acute anxiety; afraid of everything, overthinking everything, sensitive to every word that anyone spoke to me (and deeply wounded by some of those words). I felt unsafe and uncertain about my future, afraid for my children's safety and future.

afraid. unsafe. uncertain.

I've observed people I love and cherish try to help me; starting out with a plan and conviction and abruptly withdrawing. They were at a loss as to what else they could do and yet I felt so abandoned. I knew it was happening and yet I wasn't able to do anything because I couldn't speak the words out loud. Hell! I didn't have a clue what was happening to me either!

I was having flashbacks to childhood traumas, and this made me feel like my sanity was hanging in the breeze.

I changed General Practitioner, Haematologist and counsellor. I needed counselling to make these three changes - I've always believed it's better to stay with the devil you know. I have the tendency to cling to situations and experiences despite their toxicity and harmfulness, because *it is what I know* and the unknown was just way too scary for me. I've done this most of my life.

I've been seeing my current counsellor since 2016, one I interviewed over the phone before choosing to give her a go. It's been tumultuous, to say the least – unravelling, to be honest. I feel like the hideous Christmas jumper has been reduced to a tangled mess of wool and I don't know quite what to do with it.

I've felt so vulnerable and raw between sessions, and I haven't quite known what to do with myself. Most of the time, I stayed close to home and tried to keep my days simple and routine.

I've started to speak of the things that are forbidden – to unlock the secrets of my beautiful child self – to talk about the memories that keep flooding the present and leaving me confused and afraid.

ptsd: post-traumatic stress disorder

I'm no expert on this condition; other than to say I live with it daily and it's not an ideal way to live. What I do understand is that I lived through many traumas as a child and, when William (absolutely uninvited) came along, the trauma and stress associated with these times in my life was triggered. Simple as that.

When I was a child, my home felt like a warzone. I felt like I had to engage in avoiding hostile enemies, daily. I was afraid I would be killed, most of the time. I learned to become a statue and to barely breathe, at a very young age. I honed that skill to perfection by the time I reached my adult years.

I grew up with an alcoholic father who was like a hand grenade with the pin out. He was violent and unpredictable and scared me witless.

I witnessed terrifying incidents where my siblings were beaten physically by him – not to mention the emotional abuse. I won't speak any more about this here as telling this part of my story would be betraying my siblings' story. It's not all mine to tell. Please, just believe me when I say it was horrific. Occasionally, I was the child who was beaten. Always, I was afraid it was going to happen and that *I* wouldn't survive or my brother or sisters wouldn't survive.

I was sexually abused (sexual molestation) by several of my father's drinking buddies and one old paedophile who stalked me on the walk to/from school. To this day, I cannot stomach the smell of stale alcohol on anyone's breath or their skin.

I felt unsafe. I was unbelievably frightened.

The emphasis here is not really on convincing you (or me) that my story is valid or that the trauma and stress is legitimate. The emphasis is on the lingering effect of trauma and how that can just implode one day. Suddenly, everything is different and nothing is the same, yet nothing is different and everything is the same.

Years of telling myself that I am okay and that life is great and I am happy and I will have a great life, have caught up with me.

Your story lives within you and the memory of trauma exists in your very cells, long after the memories are banished from your mind. No amount of self-brainwashing will change that. Well, it didn't for me.

So here I am, trapped in my mind. My intellectual mind knows that the past has happened and I am no longer in danger of that part of my life. My emotional mind is right there in the thick of it all, terrified and unsafe. My intellectual mind knows that William (absolutely uninvited) is lying dormant in my body and I can enjoy life until that changes – and it won't change by the way. My emotional mind is terrified that William (absolutely uninvited) could become aggressive and make me very sick and lead me down the road I don't want to go down – one of chemotherapy and hospitals and ambiguous medical conversations that are just riddles, not answers and stem cell transplant and immunosuppression and nightmarish stuff.

I feel unsafe. I am unbelievably frightened.

PTSD is when life just dishes out that one thing too many times and those tenderly balanced memories/emotions come falling down around you, along with your sanity and faith and trust, and all things that you know have gotten you through before, all those social and emotional constructs that got me through the traumas, my foundations, are lying there in a pile of rubble and dust.

It's going to be a long journey I suspect, but one I am happy to be on, and each day I feel stronger in my mind and am able to manage my thoughts that little better each time.

When I process, my mind considers as many scenarios as possible, providing probable outcomes for those scenarios and this all happens in a matter of seconds, before I make a choice. It's often quite noisy in my head.

open wide the mind's caged door

I used to believe that everyone thought like I did; that all minds worked the way that mine does; that my childhood experiences were the same as other kids. I thought that because we all look similar on the outside, that what happened inside was similar too. Only now that my mind is in a bit of a mess have I had that light bulb moment and realised that this is not the case. Not everyone has a million thoughts a second or analyses the way my mind does.

When I process, my mind considers as many scenarios as possible, providing probable outcomes for those scenarios. This all happens in a matter of seconds, before I make a choice.

It's often quite noisy in my head.

Throw in PTSD and the scenarios to be considered get a whole lot scarier and not necessarily realistic. In fact, not likely realistic. And yet, nothing has ever felt so real.

Growing up in an environment that included an alcoholic, violent parent, a frightened (often unprotective) parent, and drunken sexual predators, this intense analysis was necessary for me to survive. The wrong move could, and often did, result in violence, verbal abuse and carnage.

Not to mention the trauma to the child that was me. And to my siblings. And so I came to be a control freak, finely tuned by the very quest to survive.

In many ways, my analytical strengths have helped me to be better at my work and studies. The ability to assess scenarios and weigh potential outcomes and the effect these may have on people around me, could be considered favourably in the emotional intelligence arena.

I managed life in an extraordinary way, for a long time. And I actually thought that everyone went through this intense thought process. Until William (absolutely uninvited) came along and tipped my world on its axis. And I was presented with something that is out of my control.

Despite my most desperate attempts to control William (absolutely uninvited); I have been unable to do so. I really thought that if I changed my diet and wished hard enough, prayed hard enough, filled every thought with rejection of William (absolutely uninvited), I could cure myself and William (absolutely uninvited) would disappear, be gone, like a bad dream I could wake up from.

Along came trips down memory lane, at the speed of

sound! Whenever I find myself feeling as if I am not able to control a situation (which is often) I find myself transported to a terrifying memory in my childhood and I'm not able to function as an adult; I become a small child, scared out of my wits.

Don't move, don't breathe, don't scream ... don't ... say ... a ... word. If you stay still, he won't know you're there and he won't hurt you, you won't die. Don't scream ... Don't cry ... stay still. You won't die. If you stay still, you will be invisible, you won't die.

To this day, I cry without making a sound. Now I understand why. I go into this state several times, most days.

I'm now able to understand what is happening, thanks to my therapist and ongoing gathering of knowledge about PTSD and the impact of this on the brain/psyche.

I am learning that the adult me doesn't fully disappear and, in time, I will be able to help that frightened child, soothe her and bring her home. It seems like a bloody huge mountain, that concept, right now.

But I'm up for it. No way is this going to get the better of me long term. I may be a mental health wreck a lot of the time; but my love of life and determination to get past this time in my life are solid and do not waver.

And William (absolutely uninvited), if you're listening, you can fuck off now!

I understand now why things
that move me deeply –
such as: the song,
We Are Australian
(it gets me every time);
when I witness human triumph;
personal loss; sunsets;
morning dew; hugs from my
children; random acts of
kindness – cause me to cry
tears that come from the very
core of me.

fragmented

I have an overwhelming, aching sense of abandonment.

I feel so alone. I know it's PTSD and the trauma from my very young child-self. I know it's fundamental that I be with this feeling and allow it - not that it's actually a choice for me right now; PTSD really does steam roller things such as choice and allowance.

Yet, I recognise the importance of paying attention to this feeling and understanding that for the first time in my life, I am able to connect to how my young child felt when enduring the life-shattering traumas associated with being exposed to alcoholism, physical abuse, verbal abuse and sexual abuse.

abandoned.

I was able to read a helpful book called Healing the Child Within, which explains the concept of my adult self, helping my child self to heal.

Going through the trauma I did as a child meant I was not able to develop in the same way as a child who is loved and nurtured develops.

My life started with my mother frantically grabbing me

as a young baby, from the bassinet, as my father, in a rage, grabbed the bassinet and threw it because I wouldn't stop crying. This is a story my mother told me often enough for it to be etched into my memory as the opening paragraph to the story of my life.

The inner child is described as the true me, the authentic me. And in the case of a traumatised child, co-dependence leads to the development of a series of false identities created along the way so I could exist in the world and make a life for myself.

The word **fragmented** echoes in my mind.

I have often thought of my life as having a box of masks at the front door … you know … in the same way some people have a coat rack or an umbrella box. I would choose the mask of the moment according to the environment/setting I was heading out into, slip it on, and be on my way.

I knew I was doing this, but I didn't know that it wasn't authentic or that it was co-dependency, or that my inner child was in this dark place, curled up in some dark recess, inside of me.

Until William (absolutely uninvited) came along and PTSD sent me to this dark recess, time and time again.

Intellectually, I understand the task that lay ahead of me. I'm able to draw a mind map of what needs to be done. I know that the adult me needs to acknowledge this little girl and comfort her and help to heal her.

Emotionally, this stuff scares the absolute bejeebers out of me. And PTSD sends me into flashbacks, spontaneously and without warning and oh-so frequently that I don't know what is real, most of the time.

If I encountered someone so emotionally needy, I would run a mile and, although I may look back once or twice, I would run nevertheless.

And yet here I am, confronted with helping this part of myself to somehow help this young child to overcome these overwhelming emotions and heal.

I am confronted with the truth that my inner child - my *true me*, my *authentic self* - is a terrified, abandoned child who does not want to go out into the world, who is curled up in the corner, paralysed and barely breathing.

I just don't know how to begin to heal the damage that my childhood caused to my *true me*, to my *authentic self*.

Except to just begin.

PTSD is like some warped mode of time travel; where I'm transported to the emotions of my child self, in a flashback that is triggered by something happening in real time.

I am fluctuating between not knowing what is real, raising my fist to the universe and raging that my flawless masquerades of co-dependence and mask selection at the front door have been brought to an abrupt halt; and absolute devastation that my *true me*, my *authentic self*, is so shattered and vulnerable, so traumatised and afraid.

It's as if my real-time life reached a similar parallel - feeling so shattered and vulnerable and traumatised and afraid when William (absolutely uninvited) came crashing into my life - and only then could I see that small child in the dark recess of myself. And not *unsee* her.

Abandonment is something I am experiencing now. I feel such an aching loneliness, such an enormous need for someone to rescue me, protect me and take care of me.

I am equally as horrified by this, as I am deeply saddened.

I would go as far as to say that I always saw it as a weakness in myself if I started to feel dependent on another person; I drove myself to be fiercely independent, believing that relying on another person for anything led to ultimate disappointment.

I've found it difficult to ask for help - I still do.

I have always found it difficult to *receive* - compliments, gifts, acts of kindness - I feel like I want to cry, tell off the person giving, feel weak because I couldn't meet all of my own needs, horrified that I can't just be thankful, all at the same time. Very confused and conflicted.

I am much more comfortable with giving.

I am beginning to understand why.

I understand why I protected and continue to try to protect my children to the hilt; understand where the need to do that stemmed from.

I understand now why things that move me deeply -

such as: the song *We are Australian* (it gets me every time); when I witness human triumph, personal loss, sunsets, morning dew, hugs from my children, random acts of kindness - cause me to cry tears that come from the very core of me.

I now understand why I ache when I leave a friend or a friend leaves me; when I end a phone chat; or when my children drive off - to the point that I sometimes avoid those things because I can't feel that sense of loss some days.

My journey with recovery and living with William (absolutely uninvited) goes on. I can't see the path ahead, I am forging the road I am travelling as I move along it.

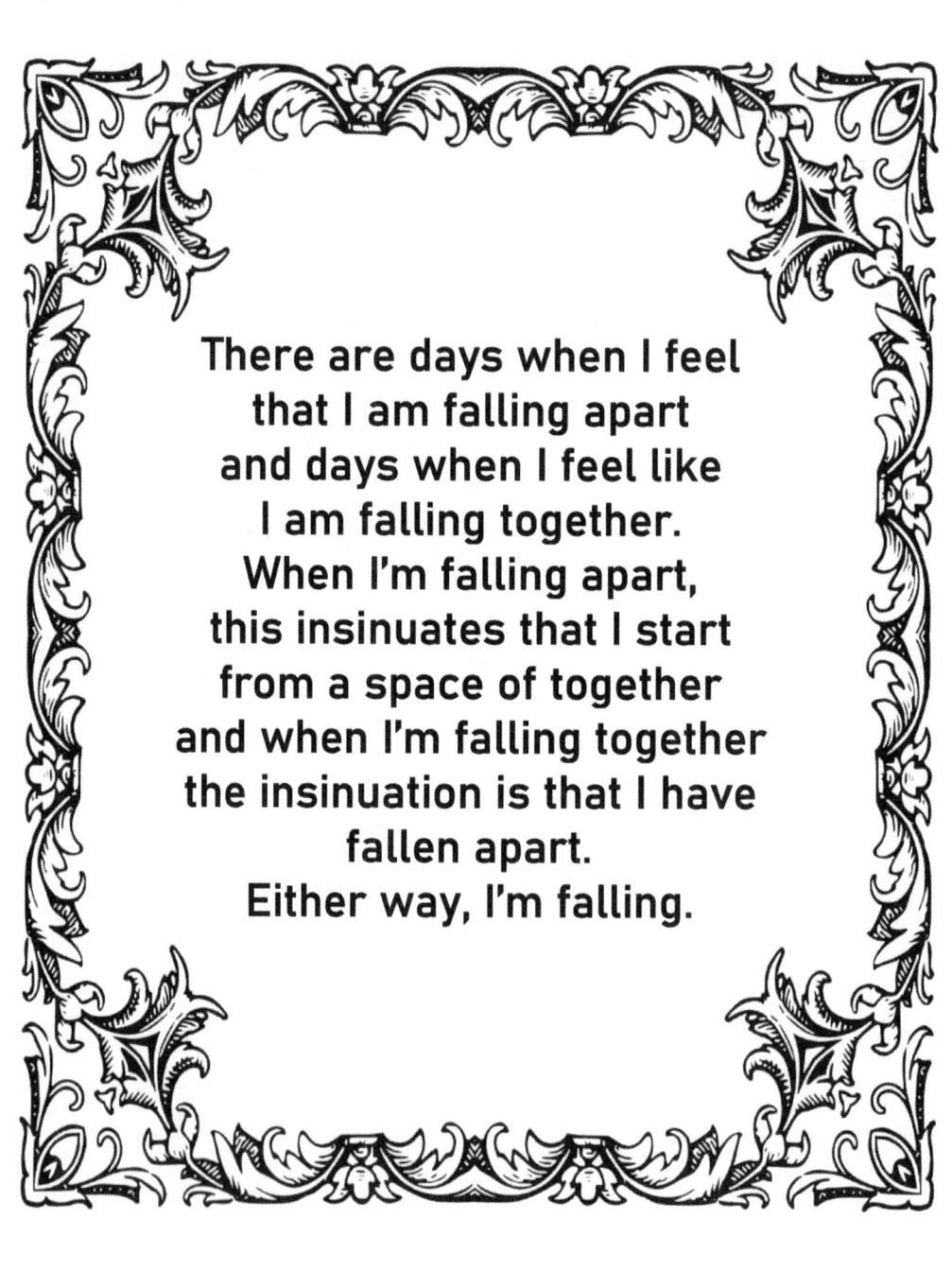

There are days when I feel
that I am falling apart
and days when I feel like
I am falling together.
When I'm falling apart,
this insinuates that I start
from a space of together
and when I'm falling together
the insinuation is that I have
fallen apart.
Either way, I'm falling.

down the rabbit hole

There are days when I feel that I am falling apart and days when I feel like I am falling together. When I'm falling apart, this insinuates that I start from a space of together and when I'm falling together the insinuation is that I have fallen apart. Either way, I'm falling.

I often liken my mental health journey to falling down the rabbit hole because I feel as though the ground went from under me and I've been trying to find solid ground ever since. Sometimes I think I've found it and, it turns out, it was only a foothold; a short reprieve, before life spiralled again.

I know this is only metaphoric and not real, but a great analogy all the same.

Anxiety and stress peaked to an all-time high in September 2016. Life threw the whole lemon tree my way. I felt my coping was slipping through my fingers like beach sand. No matter how hard I tried to take the anxiety down a notch and engage in calming techniques, I found myself very close to a nervous breakdown.

I spent a lot of time alone, with PTSD episodes triggered many times a day. I felt terrified and ashamed and so very unwell in my mind. This is when I knew, without a doubt that I needed to consider medication. The very thought of medication caused me anxiety, but fear of losing my mind was greater.

I started taking an antidepressant called Escitalopram which is more commonly known as Lexapro. At first, I felt no difference, and this was most likely because I started on a very small dose of 5mg per day. Two weeks on, an increase to 10mg started to make a difference and I started to sleep better than I have done in a very long time. Anxiety was still very high and I was having early morning panic attacks sometimes. I am now taking 20mg and find I can cope with most things that life hurls at me now.

I've been afraid of medication and resisted this for as long as I could. I truly believed that I could get on top of things without medication. It turned out that I couldn't.

Ah, but it's good to not feel stressed out all the time and to have a few giggles and smiles.

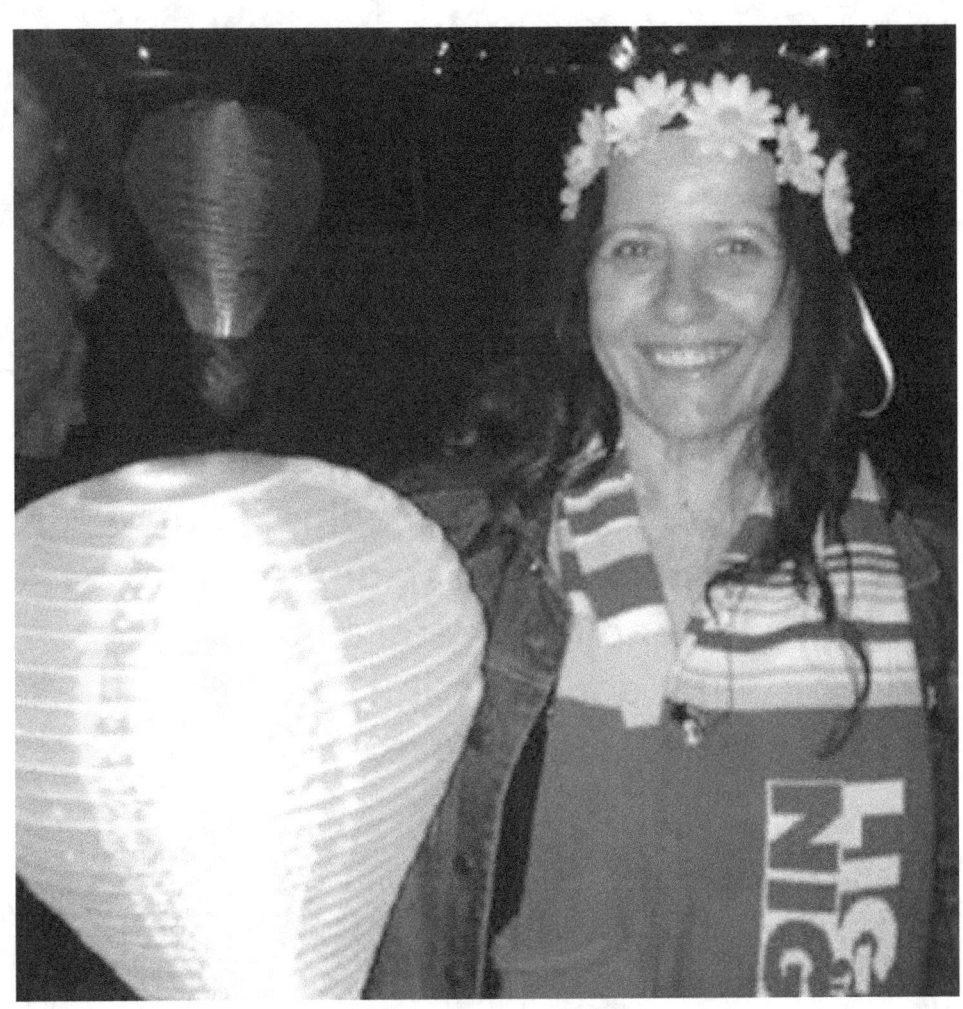

September, 2014

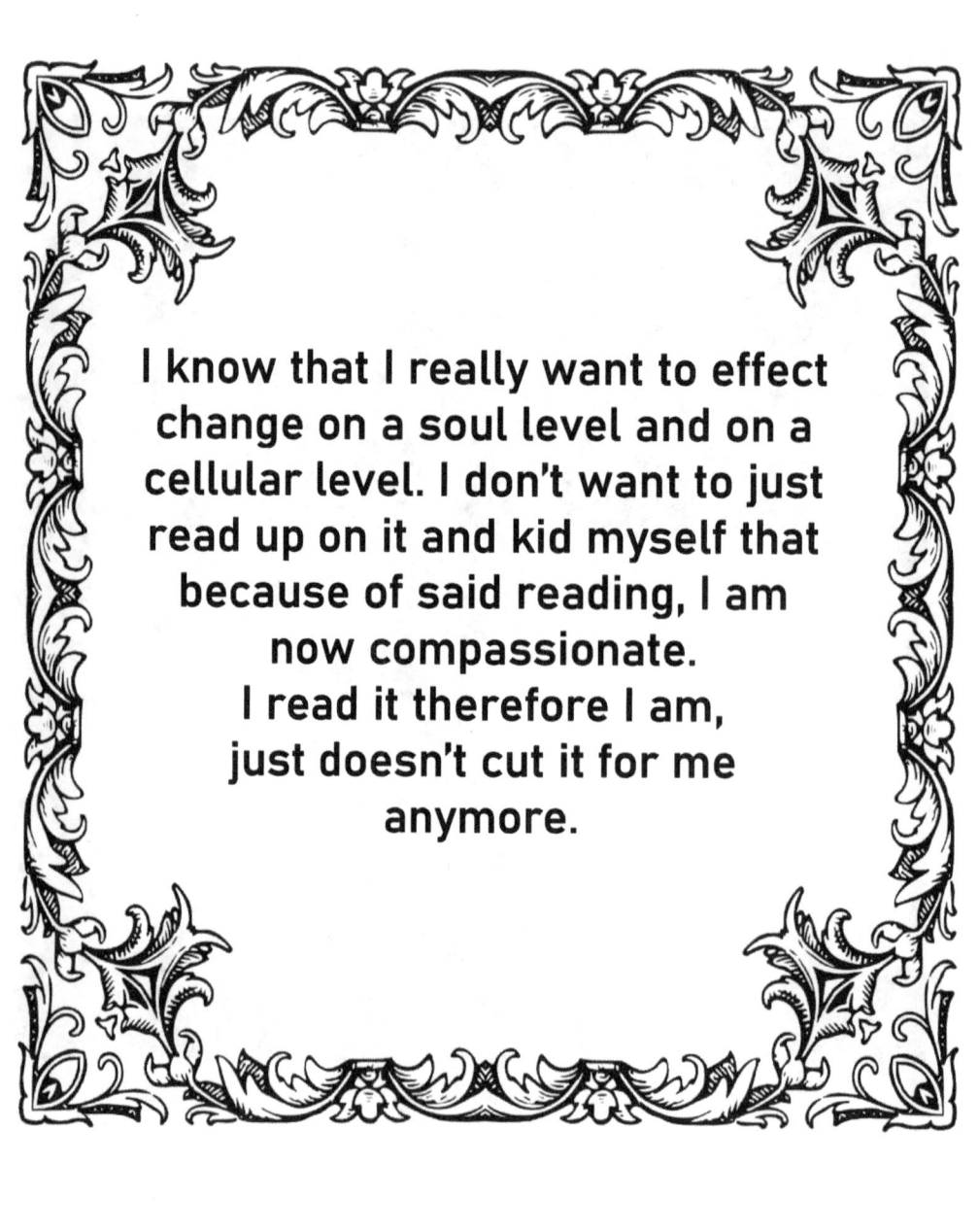

I know that I really want to effect change on a soul level and on a cellular level. I don't want to just read up on it and kid myself that because of said reading, I am now compassionate.
I read it therefore I am, just doesn't cut it for me anymore.

compassion

Compassion!! What does it mean for you? This is something I have been peeking at now for some time. I've snuck little peeks, not wanting to get caught staring and actually be a little intimidated by what I may discover, although I don't really understand why.

What have I discovered? That compassion is vital and that lack of compassion, both self and for others, goes a long way to explaining why this world is so fucked up.

Having a chronic illness gives me a sense of vision and understanding beyond what I had before William (absolutely uninvited) came along. It's like going from 2D to 3D.

The most profoundly touching experiences I have had since the 21st of March 2014, the ones that are etched in my mind and heart and continue to sustain me and nourish me, are those of compassion from another person.

The most profoundly hurtful experiences that I have had - the ones that have fed my inner critic and eaten away at my self-belief and self-esteem, that left me wondering many times how I could sustain the loss of friendship and contributed to the demise of my mental health - are those of lack of compassion; from another person and also from myself.

Some useful things I have learned along the way:

- You don't have to fix a person to help them. Most people just need someone to care, connect with them, let them know that they matter - hold space for them and stay in their lives no matter what.

- Listen to understand.

- Lack of compassion stems from lack of self-compassion - work on self-compassion and the rest will happen.

Why does this really matter? My focus on compassion came about through my commitment to mindfulness, meditation and managing severe anxiety and PTSD. My reason for feeling intimidated by this ten-letter word? I'm really looking at it for the first time.

I mean, I'm taking it seriously. I get just how important it is for me to improve my mental health and to help me live gracefully with a chronic illness.

But the biggest reason:

i cannot be authentic and i cannot be me if i cannot show myself compassion; and in doing so, learn to be compassionate toward others.

Knowing that I really want to effect change on a soul level, on a cellular level, I don't want to just read up on it and kid myself that because of said reading, I am now compassionate. I read it, therefore I am, just doesn't cut it for me anymore.

Because of therapy I am now aware of some things about myself.

I am not kind to myself.

I believe that I am weak because I cannot work. I feel like I have succumbed to having a chronic illness - as if I have a choice and I choose to have fatigue and I choose to have anxiety.

I feel lazy and worthless - and I have to add here that Centrelink (which I actually call Stinkylink in my head) makes me feel that way too. People share social media posts about welfare recipients needing to be drug tested before their hard-earned money pays those good for nothing drug addicts who collect welfare payments; those 'who could get a job but choose not to' types. I have to say I have lost immense respect for people who support that initiative. Anyways, I digress and that issue is a can of worms!

I often berate myself – "Mandy, if you could just get over this nonsense and work, you wouldn't have to worry about how you are going to pay your bills or worry that you can't help your child when he or she needs your help."

I have such grief about the loss of the person I once was, the level on which I was able to function. Such inconsolable grief. With the skills I have learned in therapy, I am able to contradict that voice and seek out the various tools I now have to combat the critical and unkind thoughts I have about myself and to understand with compassion why my mind goes to those places.

With the blind hope that, in time, and with continued practice, my first thoughts will be self-loving and kind, and there will be no more critical and unkind thoughts to be combated.

I must admit that I do get a kick out of telling that inner critic to shut the fuck up!! Like, I'm really allowed to do that, haha! Who knew?

Compassion-ability affects a person in so many ways. I am learning that people who have not been able to show me compassion are not necessarily mean or cold-hearted. It is more likely that they lack self-compassion and therefore cannot be compassionate toward other people.

WOW!

That's a far more acceptable explanation for some of the behaviours I have experienced; far more acceptable than seeing people as mean and cold-hearted - far less hurtful to me. Who would have thought it, but I actually feel compassionate toward those people.

Come closer.

I need to say something quietly.

Don't tell William (absolutely uninvited), but I like who I am becoming and what I am learning about myself since … you know … **HE showed up.**

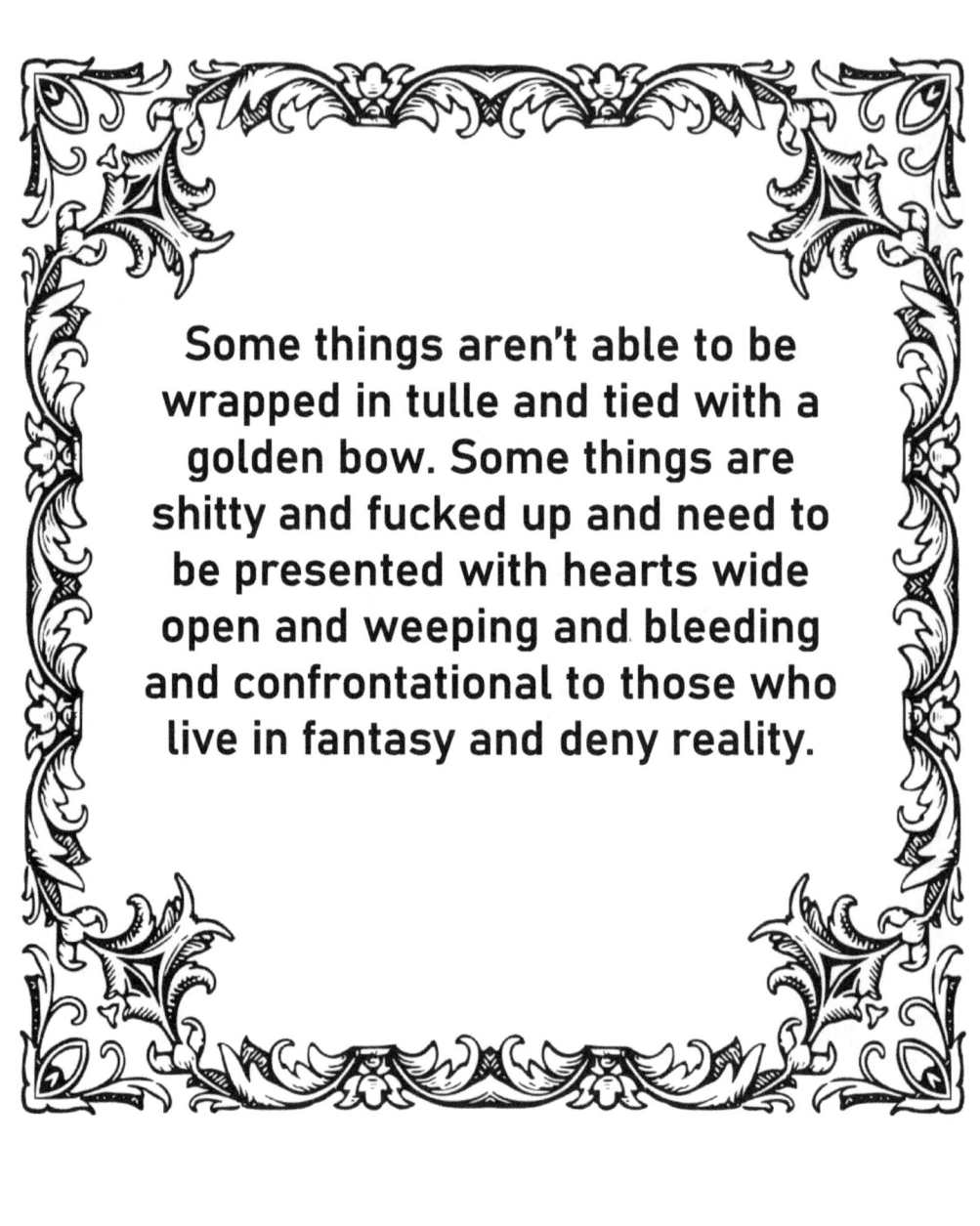

Some things aren't able to be wrapped in tulle and tied with a golden bow. Some things are shitty and fucked up and need to be presented with hearts wide open and weeping and bleeding and confrontational to those who live in fantasy and deny reality.

do you believe in fairy tales?

For most of my life, I have believed in fairy tales. I have a very romantic, fantasy-based side to me that has helped me to get through every hurdle in life … this will to believe there is something better out there for me and that I must never give up hope; that every person has good in them and every cloud is silver-lined.

I love unicorns. I believe that feathers are a message from my angels, letting me know they are around me. I can look at morning dewdrops in the garden, shining with the sun and get lost in a fantasy of fairies and a world where everything is love.

William (absolutely uninvited) came along, and I question those beliefs now. The magic I once believed in has a series of very big question marks. Or is it more the case that I have not been able to overcome William (absolutely uninvited) despite my affirmations, despite my belief in miracles, my pleas to my angels and to the universe? ... that I have been rendered still and into a state of *being* and not *doing*, with life staring me squarely in the face and my story and all its pages is laid out in front of me, every trauma jumping at me from the chapters demanding to be dealt with.

Did I choose fairy tales rather than acceptance and healing?

There are happy sentences too. They give me great comfort and help me to discover the child me. But the truth is there is more trauma than any one person should be dealt in one lifetime.

And yet, here I am, alive and breathing and discovering, my passion and curiosity for life still glowing – how fucking amazing is that? – my tenacity and endurance to survive and survive well, no matter how much this life throws at me.

The challenge for me is to learn to have one foot in reality at all times and one foot in fairy tales at all times; to believe in both, at the same time. And to define my own reality. Now that's a really hard topic for me: Is reality such a flimsy thing that it can be determined by my thoughts, my imagination, my fantasies? I used to think so. Until William (absolutely uninvited) crashed my party.

Four years on, no matter how much I have tried to create a reality for myself that embraced the disappearance of William (absolutely uninvited) and a promise to the universe that I am paying attention (and will continue to do so) that miraculous curing has not occurred. The question marks have surrounded my very existence.

There was a time when fairytales helped me to survive trauma. Sexual abuse and whispers of *our secret* into my eight-year-old ear. The lingering smell of stale alcohol that haunts me to this day. There was a time when all of this could be replaced by a pixie in the garden, bathing in the dewdrops in the land of happy.

It was much easier to be a frozen statue if my mind escaped a drunken rampage to a place of polka dot mushrooms and garden elves having picnics, or fairies flying to the moon. But it's not real, is it? We both know, it's not real. What is real? The situation is real. How I feel about it and think about it, is apparently my choice and also, apparently, not real. Just emotion. Just pain. Just joy (*insert sarcasm). This is the part I have trouble accepting. Because how I feel about situations is real to me.

Some things aren't able to be wrapped in tulle and tied with a golden bow. Some things are shitty and fucked up and need to be presented with hearts wide open and weeping and bleeding. Some things need to be confrontational to those who live in fantasy and deny reality.

We need to be made to feel uncomfortable, shocked to our core, saddened, and aware of other people's suffering and pain. We cannot be whole otherwise. And we need to damn well care.

We need to stop seeking out the company of only those who uplift us and put our arms around those who can no longer pretend, who need the warmth of our embrace and need to know that the world is a caring place that values every human being.

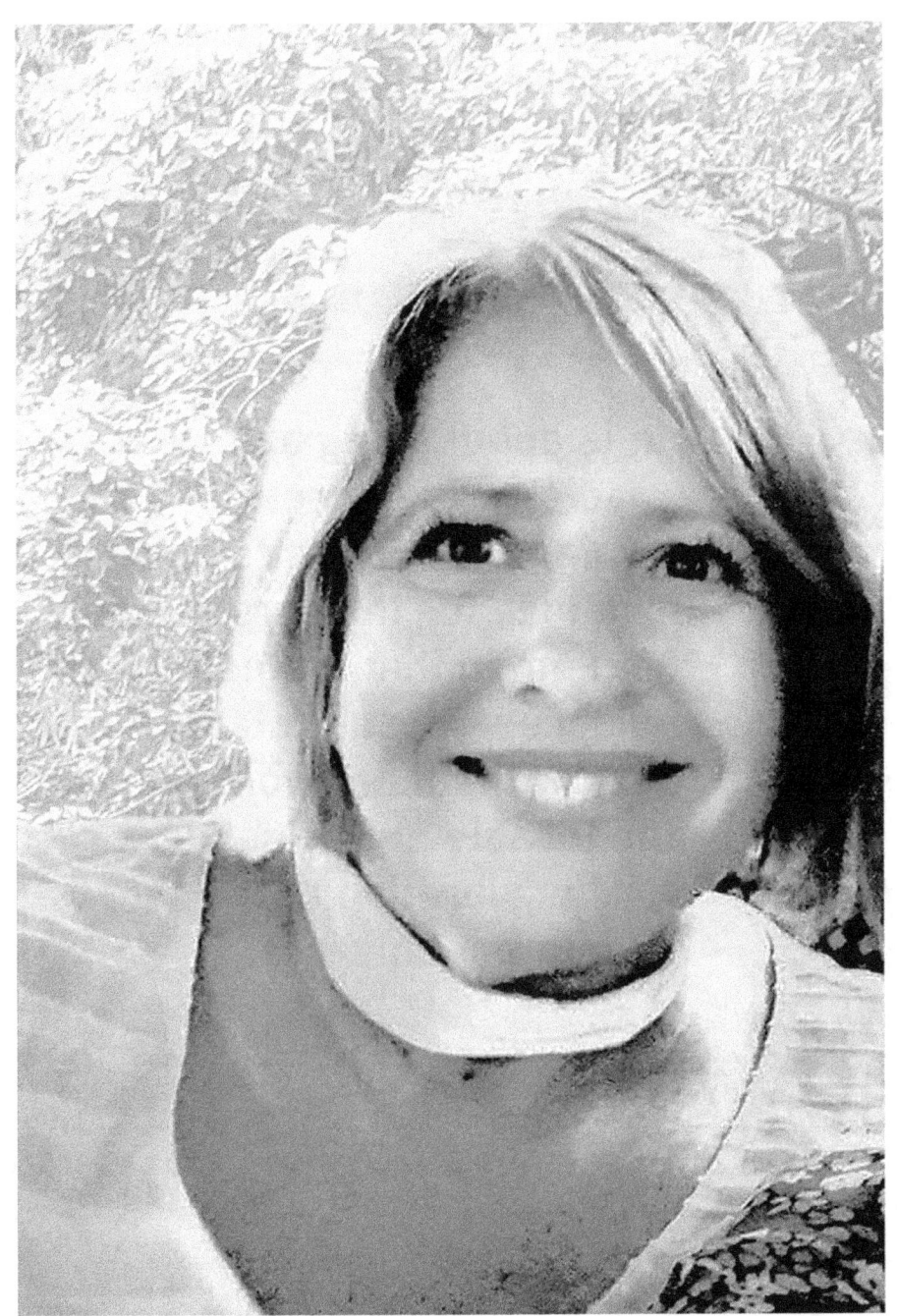

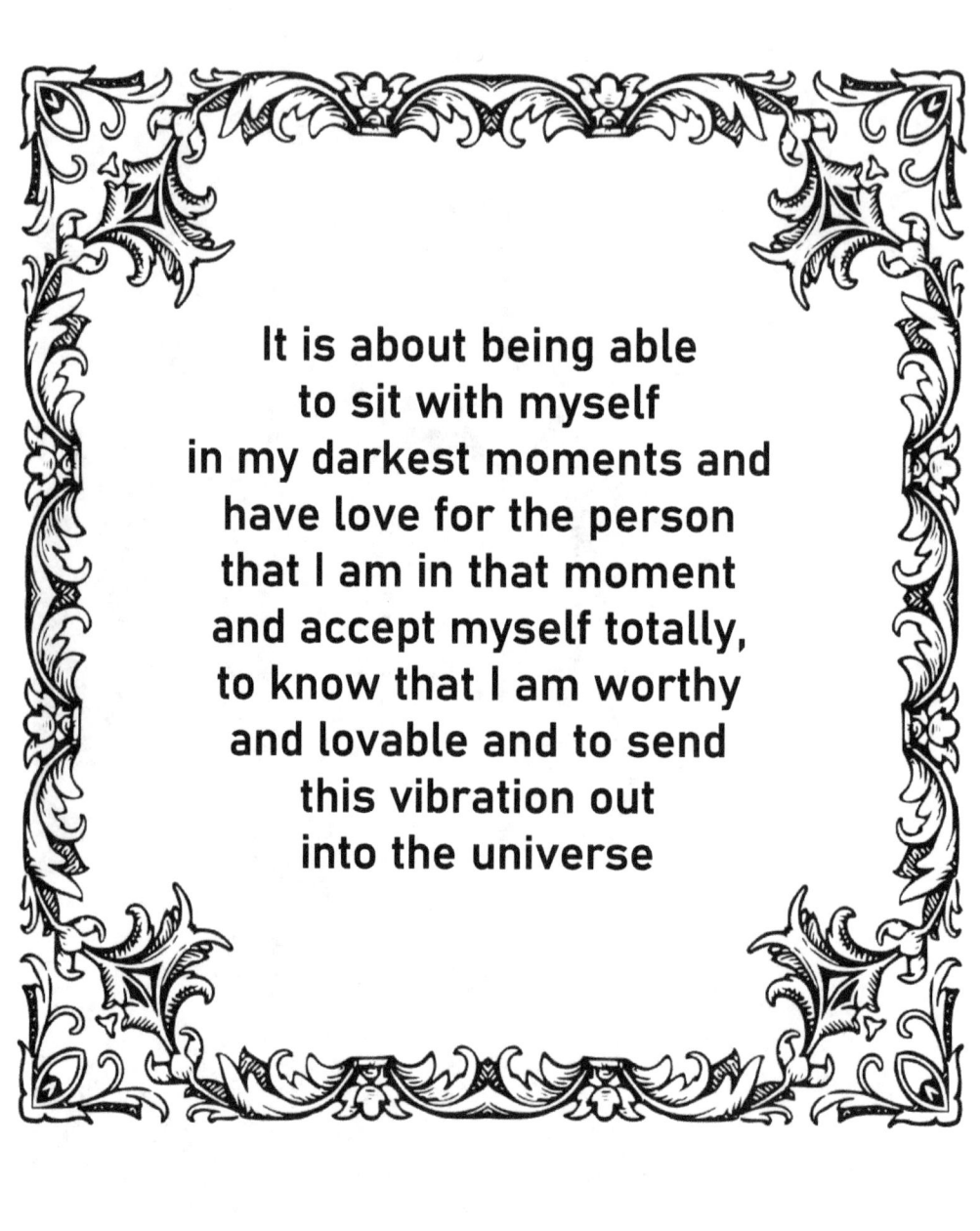

It is about being able
to sit with myself
in my darkest moments and
have love for the person
that I am in that moment
and accept myself totally,
to know that I am worthy
and lovable and to send
this vibration out
into the universe

befriending mandy

I spend a lot of time on my own, which is not uncommon for someone with a chronic illness and mental illness. Or so I'm told. Which means that the main person in my life is ME.

When your life is simplified to the extent to which mine has been, it becomes very obvious that I am not kind to myself; that I am really not my own friend. To be brutally honest, I have not forgiven myself for having cancer. It is impossible for me to accept the cancer as part of me. I think of it as something third party that I am able to reject. Which means that effectively, I cannot accept a part of myself.

Four years on from diagnosis, I am no closer to embracing this part of my life. I am simply unable to do this. I am so bloody angry.

But let's talk about my life in general and not focus on William (absolutely uninvited), because, the truth is, I have always found it difficult to be kind and supportive to myself when I need it the most. I have spent most of my life seeking validation from people, places and things outside of myself, because I didn't feel valid as a person.

I didn't grow up in an environment within which I was cherished for my uniqueness and magic, where I could play tea parties with imaginary friends, join in family laughter around the dinner table, go on family bike rides or run to my daddy at the end of his working day and be swept up in his arms.

No lullabies for me. Fucking cunt was something I heard many times a day, long before I ever knew what those words meant, although I did know it wasn't a nice thing to say because it made me feel frightened and unsafe.

Co-dependency was my area of expertise; learning what behaviour took me off the radar of an alcoholic PTSD-ridden, unpredictable, violent father; off the radar of paedophilic, drunken men who got off on fondling a defenceless and terrified child, all the while whispering in my ear about secret-keeping.

I don't profess to know what actually happened to my psyche while I was a small child, developing and growing up in a world where I was surrounded by verbal, physical and sexual abuse.

What I can tell you is that I didn't feel loved or even liked for that matter. I learned very early in life to chastise myself for my own mistakes and short-fallings, as these usually led to an abusive situation for either myself and/or my siblings. I also developed an inner critic that sounded just like my angry, drunken father.

So here I am, over 50 years old and, for the first time, trying to learn how to be kind to myself, to have respect for myself, to be my own friend.

How does this affect my life? Well, it's probably easier to ask *how does this not affect my life?* There is no part of my life that is not affected by this. Nothing is easy for me. Nothing. I am a well-honed analyst. I have a mind that simply doesn't stop.

Sometimes I choose to be alone and enjoy the solitude, usually when I am not well or when I am feeling very fatigued and low in energy or when I'm feeling too vulnerable to go out into the world outside my door. Sometimes, I would like to socialise but I often feel unable to arrange this because I feel that I am a burden to my friends - that they would prefer to not spend time with me. I have been tired and anxious for so long now that I actually don't answer when I'm asked "how are you going?" I feel that very few people really understand and I have learned to not answer as this is easier.

I feel like only a very few of the people I love actually love me and want to spend time with me.

My journey of recovery and learning to manage anxiety, depression and PTSD - which by definition is a journey of self-discovery - has brought me to a *you are not your own friend* junction.

And so I try to change the well-worn mental patterns of thought that have been with me from my earliest memories. I am trying to learn that only I can validate my existence, who I am and how I feel.

This has nothing to do with anything outside of myself. It is about my thoughts, my dreams, my passion, my integrity and my values.

It is about being able to sit with myself in my darkest moments and have love for the person that I am in that moment. It is about being able to accept myself totally; to know that I am worthy and lovable and to send this vibration out into the universe.

It is about letting go of the shame I feel about buying food from Foodbank and clothes from Good Samaritans.

It is about accepting that William (absolutely uninvited) is not really a relationship that is being forced on me, like a stalker that won't go away, but a cancer that is part of my own body - my own twisted DNA that went haywire and started to produce a protein that is foreign and poses a serious risk to my health.

It is about being able to look upon my own reflection in a mirror ... yes, that is hard on its own ... but then to say to myself *I love you, Mandy*. I'm not there yet.

It is about being able to feel pretty and not ugly and overweight and a hideous sight when I step outside my house.

It is about sitting with myself when I've banged into the door and hurt my arm; telling myself that it's okay and I will be alright, instead of berating myself for being so bloody careless and telling myself that the bruise is punishment for such carelessness.

It is about asking myself *"are you okay?"* when I'm feeling alone and wondering why I am alive in this world right now; when I am wondering what the point to my life is now. It's about being able to reassure myself at these times; to believe that it's okay to call on a friend because I am loved and cherished by others.

In all honesty, I have a way to go. It's so easy to slip into old patterns and so difficult to hold a self-intervention when I recognise that I am repeating patterns.

One step at a time, my friend.

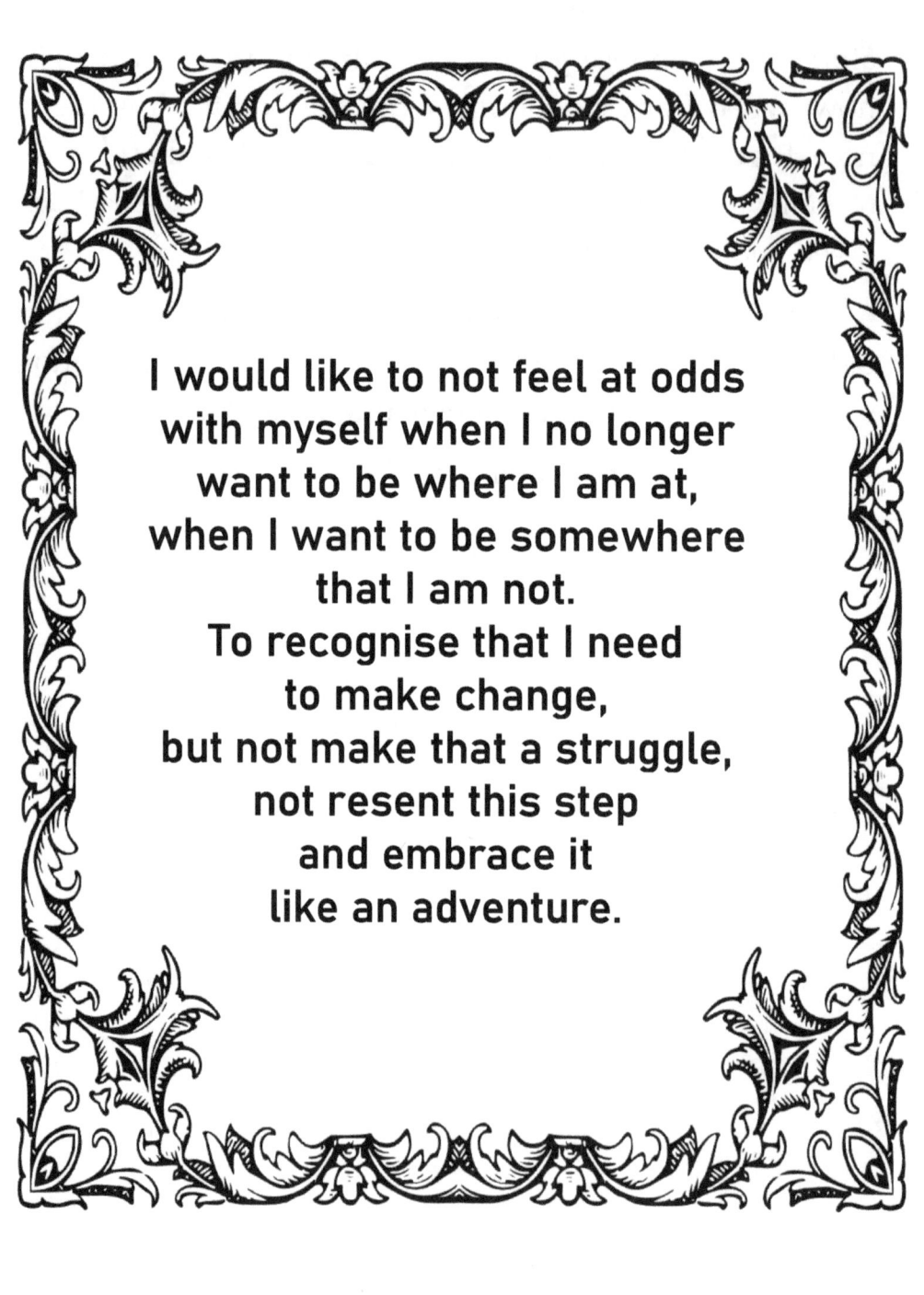

I would like to not feel at odds
with myself when I no longer
want to be where I am at,
when I want to be somewhere
that I am not.
To recognise that I need
to make change,
but not make that a struggle,
not resent this step
and embrace it
like an adventure.

the space between where i am and where i want to be

This is the space that I find so very hard to be in.

The space between where I am and where I want to be.

And yet, it is the space that I spend most of my life occupying.

This raises two issues for me:

1. Why do I always want to be somewhere other than where **I** am?

2. Why do I struggle with the in-between?

I am going to really work on these issues, as they are the

key to much of my struggle. They are central to struggle, surrender, acceptance and open-heartedness.

I really want more tranquillity and less struggle in my life. I really do.

I have not long finished reading another great book by Oriah Mountain Dreamer called *The Dance*. Part of her prose, *The Dance*, talks about the dance we choose. In the context of *life* being the *dance,* ergo: the way we choose to live our life = the way we dance.

"Don't tell me how wonderful things will be ... someday.

Show me how you can risk being completely at peace, truly okay with the way things are right now in this moment, and again in the next and the next and the next..."

This is about being truly okay with how things are in my life, right now. Not yesterday, not tomorrow. But right now.

To be able to let go of whether I like the way things are right now and to let go of the way I suffer because of this. To let go of how my body stores my dissatisfaction and resentment and to just breathe.

To accept.

To surrender.

My ability to recognise that a lack of suffering is happiness and that it lives in the space between, and where we are and where we want to be. If we would just allow it.

I was reading the chapter on *choosing a joyful dance* and I had this realisation as I read the words: the realisation that I hang onto my state of suffering when I am in the space between *where I am and where I want to be* and, in doing so, cause myself so much pain.

The concept that I could be okay with where I am at and seek inspiration from that space has piqued my curiosity and certainly challenged me to a different way of thinking; a different perception.

That I don't have to suffer to transform; that growth does not have to come from pain. I have to say that I have absolutely no idea how to do this. Would I be willing to do this if I knew how?

Absolutely yes.

I would like to not feel at odds with myself when I no longer want to be where I am at; when I want to be somewhere that I am not. I would like to recognise that I need to make a change, but not make that a struggle, not resent this step and embrace it like an adventure.

I've been in this in-between space now for six years – wanting to be free of William (absolutely uninvited) - I am coming to terms with the fact that this has not been something I can reasonably achieve, given that I have been told that Waldenstroms Macroglobulinaemia is incurable.

Where I would like to be in my life is: financially secure and able to live in such a way that I don't have to work and can make maintaining my physical and mental health my highest priority.

I realise things need to be done if I am to get to where I want to be.

I tried for three years to claim a Disability Support Pension and, after three claims, I achieved this. I received approval for my claim on Total and Permanent Disability insurance, which has been paid into my superannuation. Financial struggle dissipated in a cloud of smoke!

I am able to maintain health with a lifestyle that doesn't involve the stress of working and enables me to access various calming and healing therapies.

I'm able to walk the beach at any time and for as long as I need to. I know that this is the way it is meant to be.

Reflecting on where I was six years ago and where I am today (although I am not yet where I want to be), I understand the need for the in-between. I now understand the in-between allows time for me to take the steps that I have needed to take.

It's like a trapeze: you can only let go when you have the next swing lined up and within your grasp.

Another excerpt from the book *The Dance* that laps at my feet like the ocean - it's written on the front cover and captivated me instantly!

"What if the question is not why I am so infrequently the person I really want to be, but why do I so infrequently want to be the person I really am?"

Just reading this quiets my internal struggle to be

someone other than who I really am. It calms me. It *really* calms me.

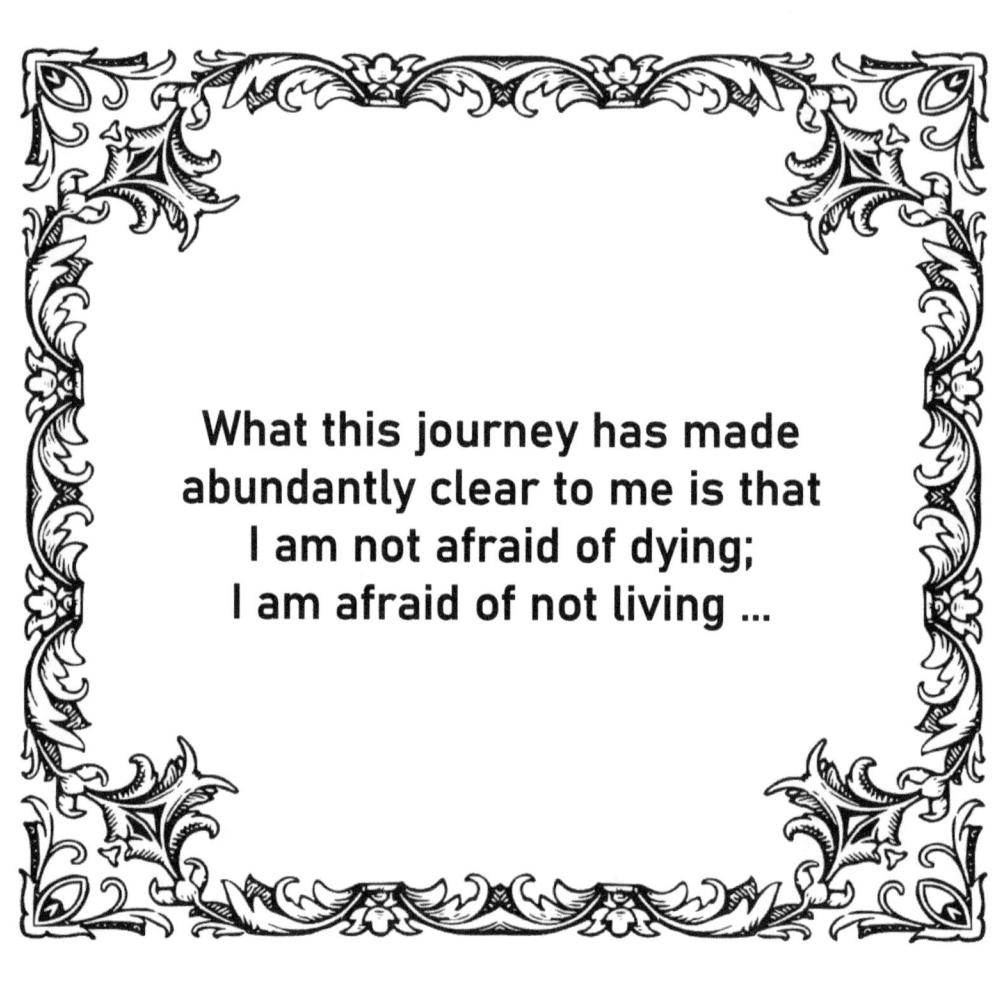

What this journey has made
abundantly clear to me is that
I am not afraid of dying;
I am afraid of not living ...

a mountain with a view

I woke late this morning. The sun was beaming off the water in the birdbath and reflecting on the ceiling of my bedroom. I was completely mesmerised and so content in that moment. Who knew that I could reach this point in my life? Seriously? I had completely lost faith in the idea that I could feel so joyful and peaceful.

Yet, here I am.

I've climbed a mountain and I'm enjoying the view. I'm really not sure when I reached the summit or that this is the summit. I've had my head down and bum up, duelling with Centrelink, dodging William (absolutely uninvited) at every opportunity, and practising mindfulness that I've been looking at the breeze on the leaves and not the whole tree.

Suddenly, I look around me and I'm totally amazed that I'm no longer climbing a mountain! I did a 360 degree spin, arms wide and giddy with excitement, oh, and not to be overlooked: my feet are firmly planted on the ground. I'm just going to sit here and take in every bit of beauty and listen to the whispers of the wind.

The sunsets and sunrises are spectacular by the way.

I don't know what the future holds for me. None of us do. But one thing you can be sure of is I'll be enjoying each moment as it arrives.

What this journey has made abundantly clear to me is that I am not afraid of dying; I am afraid of not living.

I haven't been able to look to the future since William (absolutely uninvited) came crashing into my life. Until now, that is. I'm not exactly the sky-diving type, I don't seek out adrenalin, but I'm pretty damn certain I have some very exciting times ahead.

But, then, that's another story that will inevitably unfold.

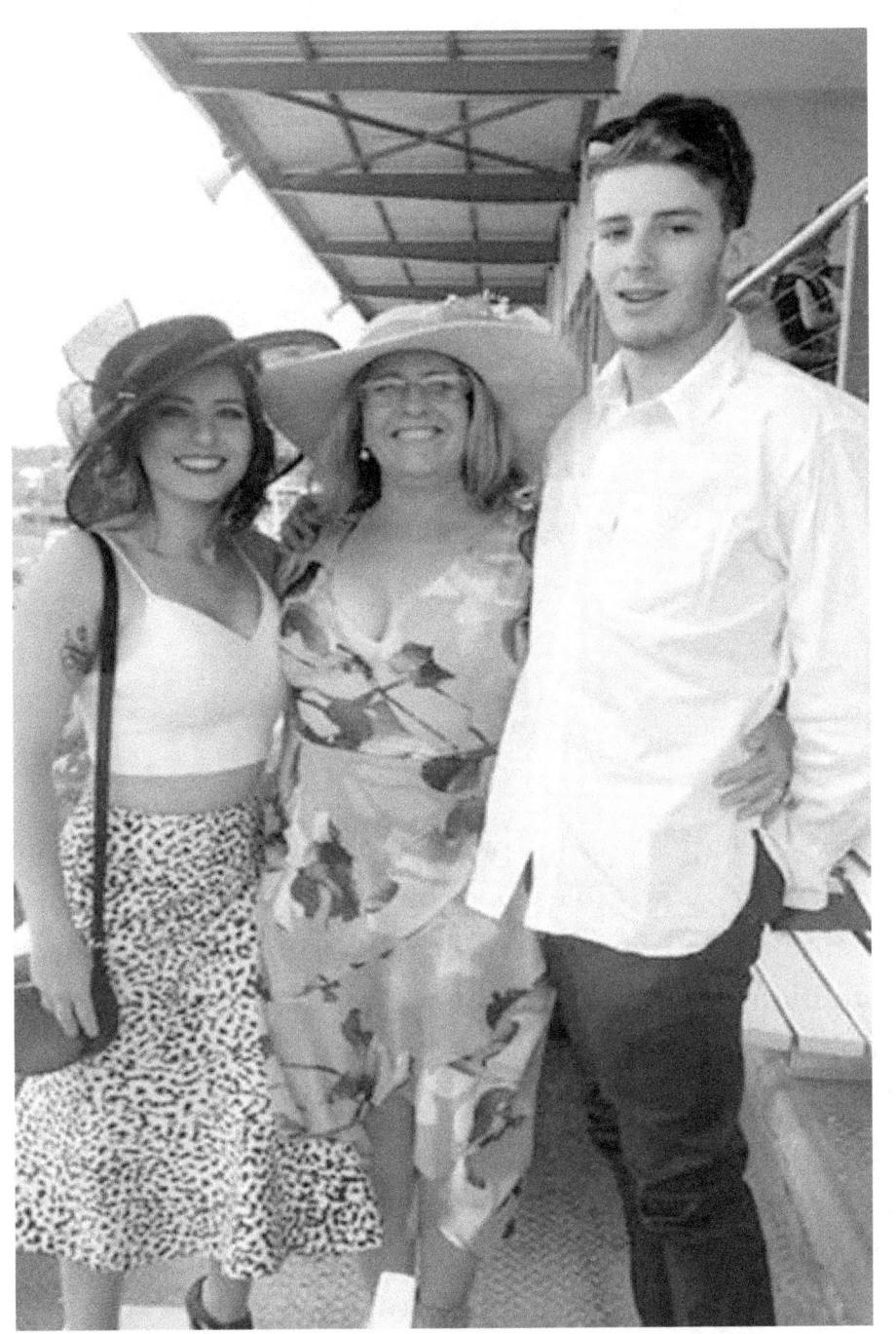

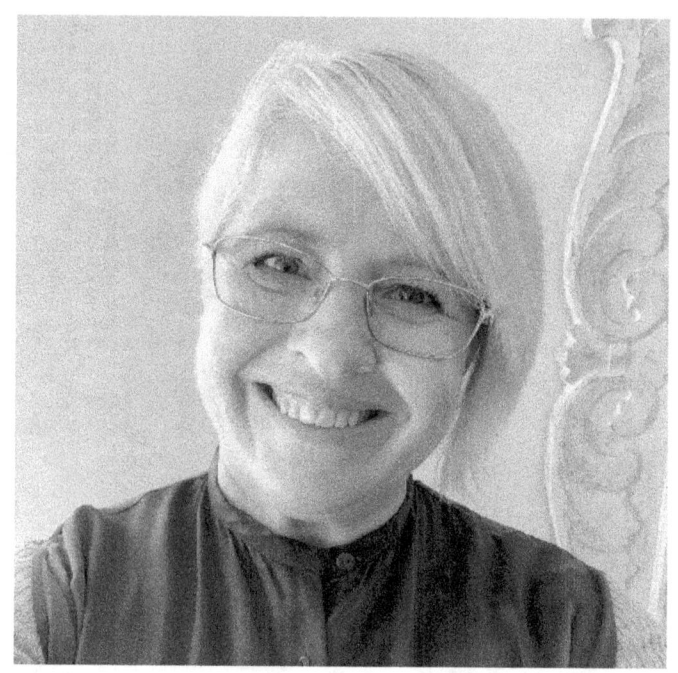

About the Author

Mandy Duggan is a published author, blogger and songwriter who lives in the south-west of Western Australia. Retirement in 2015 due to a chronic health condition was life-changing and Mandy wrote this, her first book, as a powerful healing tool for herself and readers. Mandy felt compelled to share her own story; if her journey could help just one person then it made it worthwhile. Becoming a published author has also created the opportunity for Mandy to give inspirational talks which have been an amazing experience.

www.ingramcontent.com/pod-product-compliance
Lightning Source LLC
Chambersburg PA
CBHW082104280426

43661CB00089B/854